"In this practical, concise, and sophisticated new book, Barish provides an integrative approach to child psychotherapy based upon a wonderful synthesis of the latest developments in emotion theory and research, infant developmental research, psychoanalytic theory, and cognitive approaches. By emphasizing the fundamental role played by emotion regulation in both healthy functioning and the therapeutic process, he provides a coherent theoretical framework that illuminates the way in which a range of different therapeutic interventions operate. Conceptualizing play therapy as a vehicle for facilitating emotion regulation and the renegotiation of self-other relationships, Barish provides a theoretically stimulating and clinically rich guide that will be appreciated by clinicians of all orientations."

—*Jeremy D. Safran, Ph.D., Professor and Director of Clinical Psychology, New School for Social Research, and author of* Negotiating the Therapeutic Alliance: A Relational Treatment Guide

"Dr. Barish has written an eloquent book for the use of emotions as a central component in psychotherapy with young children and with their families. His main premise, that children develop the capacity to recover or 'bounce back' from frustrations and disappointments in childhood, is clearly explained through his presentations of case material. The beginning of the book offers a clear theoretical foundation for his work, emphasizing the variety of emotions humans experience. Each emotion is carefully discussed, with examples from his practice demonstrating how he handled a particular negative emotion of a troubled child, and then how he used the emotion as a stepping stone to open the way for healing. The practical suggestions for parents and for teachers at the end of the book add to the richness of his discourse."

—*Dorothy Singer, Senior Research Associate, Yale Child Study Center, and co-editor of* Play = Learning: How Play Motivates and Enhances Children's Cognitive and Social-Emotional Growth

"This is a most impressive, comprehensive, and authoritative contribution towards understanding both the development of emotions in children as well as the child's lived experience of emotions as 'signals to ourselves and to others.' Dr. Barish's perspective focuses considerable attention on reparative experiences, which he argues become determinative elements in identity formation and character structure. Accordingly, he stresses the crucial but underappreciated therapeutic value of empathic listening and its role in helping children develop the capacity for age-appropriate affect-regulation. This is a must-read book for both experienced and beginning child psychotherapists."

—*Kirkland C. Vaughans, Ph.D., Editor,* Journal of Infant, Child, and Adolescent Psychotherapy

"This book is a gem: practical, wise, and scholarly. Dr. Barish integrates the best of a psychodynamically informed perspective with recent research-based findings from the neurosciences, attachment research, and cognitive-behaviorally as well as systemically informed perspectives. I wish I could have read this book when I was beginning my clinical work."

—*Jonathan Cohen, Ph.D., President, Center for Social and Emotional Education, and co-author of* Making Your School Safe: Strategies to Protect Children and Promote Learning

"An insightful, integrative, and clinically sensitive book that will help students and professionals of all major theoretical orientations appreciate the value of emotions and emotion theory in the practice of child psychotherapy. Barish presents a rich theoretical and conceptual framework in which to understand and treat diverse childhood disorders. This book comes at a particularly important time, when empirical support for various treatments is growing dramatically, and when the field is looking for developmentally sensitive interventions that not only incorporate emotion theory but also possess evidence that they actually work. The approach espoused in this book, although not fully tested at this time, will surely help set the stage for thoughtful review and appraisal of such interventions. It is a must-read for all serious students of child psychotherapy."

—*Thomas H. Ollendick, Ph.D., University Distinguished Professor and Director, Child Study Center, Virginia Polytechnic Institute and State University*

"Dr. Barish has done the impossible: he's written a practical, engrossing, meticulously documented and researched, authoritative, brief, and innovative book on psychotherapy with children. All clinicians who work with children will love this book, and they will rejoice in how much they learn in so few pages! A triumph!"

—*Edward Hallowell, M.D., author of* The Childhood Roots of Adult Happiness, Crazy Busy, Delivered from Distraction, *and other books*

Emotions in Child Psychotherapy

An Integrative Framework

KENNETH BARISH, PH.D.

OXFORD
UNIVERSITY PRESS
2009

OXFORD
UNIVERSITY PRESS

Oxford University Press, Inc., publishes works that further
Oxford University's objective of excellence
in research, scholarship, and education.

Oxford New York
Auckland Cape Town Dar es Salaam Hong Kong Karachi
Kuala Lumpur Madrid Melbourne Mexico City Nairobi
New Delhi Shanghai Taipei Toronto

With offices in
Argentina Austria Brazil Chile Czech Republic France Greece
Guatemala Hungary Italy Japan Poland Portugal Singapore
South Korea Switzerland Thailand Turkey Ukraine Vietnam

Published by Oxford University Press, Inc.
198 Madison Avenue, New York, New York 10016
www.oup.com

Oxford is a registered trademark of Oxford University Press.

Library of Congress Cataloging-in-Publication Data

Barish, Kenneth.
Emotions in child psychotherapy : an integrative framework / Kenneth Barish.
p. cm.
Includes bibliographical references.
ISBN 978-0-19-536686-0
1. Child psychotherapy. 2. Emotions. I. Title.
RJ504.B33 2009
618.92'8914—dc22 2008041071

This book is dedicated to the memory of my parents—Bernard and Min Barish—whose warmth and generosity survives as an inspiration in the lives of their children and grandchildren. And, with love and gratitude, to Harriet, Rachel, and Dan—what it's all about.

Contents

Acknowledgments

I would like to express my appreciation to the many colleagues, friends, and family members who have supported me in the course of writing this book:

To the faculties of the Westchester Center for the Study of Psychoanalysis and Psychotherapy, the William Alanson White Institute Child and Adolescent Psychotherapy Training Program, and the Department of Psychiatry, Weill Medical College, for offering me the opportunity to teach and supervise talented students.

To colleagues and family members who generously read earlier versions of the book and offered helpful criticism: Dan Barish, Harriet Barish, Rachel Barish, Jane Bloomgarden, Elizabeth Mayer, Eric Mendelsohn, David Newman, James Rembar, Thomas Schreiber, Paul Siegel, and anonymous reviewers of my proposal and manuscript.

To the members of my current Study Groups, colleagues with whom I have shared ideas over many years: David Aftergood, Laurence Baker, Laura Bartels, Judy Berenson, David Breindel, Diane Caspe, I. Barry Lorinstein, Cynthia Mintz, Martin Mintz, John Turtz, and Arnold Zinman. For the past decade, I have benefited especially from the scholarship and teaching of Arnold Richards, who has consistently encouraged the development of my ideas even when they have differed from his own.

To my secretary, Bobbie Gallagher, for 20 years of assistance with all aspects of my practice, teaching, and writing.

To Marcia Miller, librarian of New York-Presbyterian Hospital, Westchester Division. Without Marcia's help, I would still be searching through stacks of library books and this volume would not yet be written.

To Sarah Harrington, my editor at OUP, for thoughtful readings and constructive criticism of my manuscript at different stages in its development.

To Cindy Hyden, who offered encouragement and wise advice as I was beginning this project.

And, finally, to my friend Mary Caldwell, for 60 years of friendship and support to four generations of the Barish family.

Emotions in Child Psychotherapy

Introduction: Why Emotion?

Over the past two decades, the theory and practice of child psychotherapy have been gradually, but radically, transformed. A new research discipline—developmental psychopathology—has emerged (Cicchetti and Cohen, 2006; Toth and Cicchetti, 1999) and the classical psychodynamic model of inner conflict, although still relevant, now occupies a smaller place in our understanding of the psychological development of the child. Evidence-based cognitive and behavioral treatments, especially for children with anxiety (Kendall, Aschenbrand, and Hudson, 2003), depression (Stark et al., 2008), and behavioral disorders (Kazdin, 2005; Webster-Stratton and Reid, 2003) have been developed; the contribution of biological factors in the etiology of childhood disorders is now widely recognized; and child therapists of all schools have come to appreciate the critical role of parents in the therapeutic process.

Still, despite these salutary changes in theory and practice, essential questions remain, both about the origins and course of pathological development in childhood and about the mechanisms of therapeutic change (Kazdin, 2000). In our daily practice, all of us who work with children are presented complex clinical problems that require comprehensive diagnostic evaluation and a multifaceted approach to treatment. It is perhaps a truism—but perhaps not—that no single theory of pathological development adequately describes the complex interplay of etiological factors—biological vulnerability, family relationships, and inner conflict—that determine a child's presenting problems; and that no single therapeutic model is adequate to successfully treat the diversity of clinical problems we encounter in daily practice—or even in a single case.

An Integrative Framework

This book is offered as a contribution to the clinical theory and technique of child psychotherapy. I will present an integrative framework for therapeutic work with children and families, based on a contemporary understanding of the child's emotional experience. Emotions, of course, have been a central concern of child therapists from the beginning, especially in the humanistic and psychodynamic traditions of child therapy, but also, in some respects, in cognitive-behavioral treatments as well. In recent years, dysregulation of emotion has been increasingly recognized, by all schools, as a core feature of many forms of child and adolescent psychopathology.

When talking about emotions, it is difficult to avoid saying things that are not already commonly known, or even, common sense. Recent advances in the psychology and neuroscience of emotions, however (see, for example, Barrett and Campos, 1987; Barrett, 1998; Fischer, Shaver, and Carnochan, 1990; Fredrickson, 1998; Frijda, 2000; 2007; Izard, 1991; Panksepp, 1998), offer a broader understanding of the child's emotions and emotional development—the adaptive biological functions of emotions and the processes of appraisal, subjective experience, and action readiness that link thought, feeling, and behavior. In the course of this book, I will attempt to demonstrate how a systematic focus on the child's emotions, especially when we include the motivating and sustaining role of positive emotions, provides a revised perspective on optimal and pathological development in childhood, new understandings of all phases of the therapeutic process, and effective strategies for resolving some of our most persistent clinical problems.

A Language of Emotion

The essential language of child therapy is a language of emotions. Whether they are engaged in play or talk, the child's affects are central to a clinical dialogue with children. It is principally through the therapist's empathic recognition and responsiveness to the child's emotions that children feel known (Sander, 2002) and understood, and through the child's expression of emotion that we know the child is engaged with us in meaningful interaction. And, I believe, changes in the child's experience of emotions—increased expression of positive emotions and increased tolerance for, and recovery from, painful feelings—underlies all lasting behavioral improvement. Our appreciation of the child's emotions, the conditions that evoke and sustain them, what the child's feelings are "about"—the child's needs, "projects" (Nussbaum, 2001), and "concerns" (Frijda, 2007)—and then, the complex elaboration of the child's emotions in fantasy, attitudes, and behavior, constitutes the starting point of our therapeutic efforts and a revised or expanded "therapeutic core purpose" (Shapiro and Esman, 1985).

Plan of the Book

I begin with a review of some widely accepted principles regarding the nature of emotions and an evolutionary-functional analysis of some representative emotions—interest, shame and pride, anxiety, anger, and sadness—that are essential, but often underappreciated, in therapeutic work with children. This discussion, at first glance, may seem remote from everyday clinical practice. Along the way, I will illustrate how a functional understanding of these emotions reveals some familiar, but also some surprising and helpful, insights—about their evolutionary origins and current adaptive functions, and their importance in the life of the developing child.

I then present an emotion-based theory of optimal and pathological development in childhood. In this model, emotional health is based on a predominance of positive emotions and positive expectations. In health, children are exuberant and they want to "do things." In optimal development, the child develops the capacity to quickly recover, or "bounce back," from the inevitable frustrations and disappointments of childhood. This essential maturational process—the child's ability to restore a positive sense of himself and others, what we call emotional *resilience*—is, in my view, the critical variable in the psychological health of the child.

In pathological development, painful emotions *remain active* in the mind of the child. Some failure of emotional resilience—a child's inability to bounce back from emotional injury and distress—whether manifest as aggressive and oppositional behavior or as persistent avoidance and withdrawal—is invariably present in the lives of troubled children. Painful affects—bad feelings the child cannot "get rid of" (and then, maladaptive ways of coping with these feelings)—have come to dominate the child's "emotional landscape" (Lewis and Douglas, 1998). When parents consult us about their children, children have become demoralized and angry, and the child's emotional life is characterized by qualities of urgency and inflexibility. Children—and families—are increasingly "stuck"—locked in destructive patterns of emotional response, vicious cycles of interaction that sustain or exacerbate the child's negative emotions, attitudes, and behaviors.

Based on this understanding of optimal and pathological development, I present a multi-dimensional approach to therapeutic work with children and families. All phases of the therapeutic work, beginning with our initial engagement of the child and continuing—when we convey empathic understanding, when we challenge or "nudge" children toward more active engagement with others and more mature forms of relatedness, and when we attempt to ameliorate destructive patterns of parent-child interactions—are guided by an effort to promote emotional resilience: to arrest the spread of malignant events in the mind of the child, strengthen the child's expectation of affirming responsiveness, and restore more optimistic expectations about his future.

* * *

This therapeutic model differs in significant respects from both classical and contemporary psychodynamic approaches to child therapy. My understanding of psychological development, however, remains fundamentally psychodynamic. Among our various developmental models, psychodynamic theory best describes the events that seem to me most critical to the psychological growth and well-being of the child—the importance, for example, of empathy and of parental pride. Psychodynamic theory also best describes the *fate* of the child's emotions—the child's efforts to cope with painful feelings and how emotions are ultimately expressed in the child's attitudes and behavior, for example, in disguised expressions of anger and defiance.

The contemporary child therapist, however, faces a quandary. Psychodynamic approaches to child therapy have not received significant empirical support (Fonagy et al., 2002). Cognitive and behavioral techniques—therapeutic interventions that foster positive parenting, reduce coercive interactions, alter pessimistic thinking, and promote active problem-solving—have been proven to be useful in the treatment of many children and families. But these techniques still do not reach many other angry, withdrawn, and resistant children. And, in my view, cognitive and behavioral theories do not tell us enough about what matters most to children—and to many parents.

A systematic focus on the child's emotions helps solve this theoretical and practical dilemma. I will offer a developmental and therapeutic framework that allows us to retain essential contributions of humanistic and psychodynamic theory—enduring ideas that are helpful to *all* children and families—and also make use of the active behavioral and problem-solving interventions that are of proven value to many.

Emotions are the common ground of contemporary child psychotherapy. Emotion is our common language in talking with children and improved emotion regulation—or emotional resilience—is our common therapeutic goal. And emotions are not just "feelings"—our emotions are biologically adaptive, "complex functional wholes" (Fischer et al., 1990). From a contemporary perspective, distinctions between affect, cognition, and behavior are often arbitrary: thinking influences feeling, and feeling organizes and directs thought and action.

* * *

The therapeutic strategies I offer in this book apply primarily to the treatment of school-age children and early adolescents. Many of the techniques I will discuss are also helpful to preschool children, and the pathogenic pathways I will describe—vicious cycles of demoralization and defiance—are readily observable in troubled adolescents. Therapeutic interventions with both very young children and with adolescents, however, involve many unique problems and require separate consideration.

My goals for this book are both theoretical and practical. I have been encouraged, in the course of presenting these ideas in workshops and lectures to different groups of clinicians, by the positive response of even experienced therapists, who report some new perspective or openness in their work, with good results. But the book is addressed principally to students. My students, trained in different therapeutic models, frequently express the need for an integrative approach to the complex clinical problems they encounter. I hope that the ideas and therapeutic recommendations I present will encourage beginning child therapists to think broadly about the problems of behavior and emotional development presented to them in clinical practice and help get them started—on the right track—in their work with children and families.

Part I

Normal and Pathological Development in Childhood

1

Emotions and Emotional Development

Emotions: Basic Tenets

I begin, in this chapter, with a selective review of recent theory and research on the nature of emotions and a discussion of several emotions that are particularly important in clinical work with children. I will briefly describe some widely accepted principles that have special relevance to our understanding of both normal and pathological child development and the therapeutic process.

There are, of course, continuing controversies and unsolved problems in the study of human emotions and in our understanding of particular emotions. In recent decades, however, a consensus has emerged among emotion theorists. This understanding, most often referred to as a "functionalist" approach, highlights the adaptive (as opposed to disruptive) function of emotion.[1] In this model, emotions are understood as multicomponent processes, "complex functional wholes" (Fischer, Shaver, and Carnochan, 1990), that organize thought and action in the service of goals or "concerns" (Frijda, 2000; 2007) essential to our physical survival and psychological well-being. Emotions focus our attention, direct our thought and imagination, evoke memories, and prepare us for action. A child's recurring emotional experiences establish the basic structures of her character and adaptation to life—the memories, expectations, and response tendencies that guide her future thought and behavior.[2]

Each emotion (or emotion family) consists of a characteristic appraisal or "appreciation" of events (Barrett and Campos, 1987), a unique subjective experience (our "feelings"), a characteristic pattern of physiological activity, typical facial, postural, and vocal expressions, and a characteristic action tendency or action disposition. It is important to keep in mind, especially when considering the influence of emotions on the development of character and personality, that the appraisals and subjective experiences associated with any emotion may have both conscious and non-conscious aspects, and that action tendencies may be expressed as thoughts, attitudes, and fantasy, not only in overt behavior.

Emotions are signals to ourselves and to others—"a system of social communication" (Izard, 1991), evoked by concerns (Frijda, 2007). The observable, expressive aspects of emotions (a smile or cry, an angry or submissive posture, a look of disgust) evolved as signals to others and have the general purpose of evoking a response from others. The expression of positive emotions (for example, an infant's smiles) are signals of safety that initiate and sustain social engagement. The conscious, or experiential, aspect of emotions—our feelings—serve as signals to ourselves—an evolved mechanism that makes possible rapid evaluation and action in response to dangers and opportunities. "Emotional sensitivity represents a very fundamental and general process of evaluation . . . signaling events that are relevant to the individual's well-being or concerns to the cognitive and action systems" (Frijda, 1994, p. 113).[3] Emotions, then, are communications—to others and to ourselves—that something is right or that something is wrong. This communicative function is inherent in the nature of emotion; emotions are signals that are meant to be perceived.

Every emotion is associated with a characteristic action tendency or action disposition. Interest, for example, motivates exploration; anger motivates attack; fear motivates escape; shame motivates concealment. Panksepp (1998) has argued that our basic human emotions originated as instinctual action systems, shared by all mammals. Action dispositions are the most readily modifiable—and therefore the most culturally diverse—component of an emotion. General response tendencies, including thoughts and fantasies, are probably invariant for each emotion; these general action dispositions, however, are "acted on and often transformed by cultural learning" (Levenson, 1994, p. 125).

A contemporary functionalist understanding of emotions includes several additional important principles. The process of appraisal that elicits an emotional response includes an appraisal of the person's coping potential (Fischer, Shaver, and Carnochan, 1990; Gross and Thompson, 2007). This principle is perhaps most apparent when we consider our experience of anxiety or fear, but is also true of other emotions, for example, interest, sadness, anger, and shame. The quality or intensity of an emotion we experience depends to a considerable extent on our assessment of our capacity to cope with the challenge presented, whether this is a situation of threat (as in our experience of fear or anxiety) or an opportunity (as in our experience of interest). It is likely that a conscious or unconscious feeling (appraisal) of helplessness or futility (for example, a child's feeling that "there is nothing I can do about this") intensifies the experience of negative emotions; a feeling of futility may also attenuate (or limit the range of circumstances that will evoke) the experience of positive emotions, for example, interest, excitement, and joy.

In everyday experience, we tend to regard emotions as frequent, but short-lived, events. Although this is in some sense true—we are not continuously angry or joyful—Izard and Ackerman (2000) suggest that "emotions influence personality functioning continuously, not just episodically" and that "some emotion at some level of intensity is continuously present in consciousness." Izard and Ackerman refer to this idea as the "Principle of Continuous Influence" (p. 261). Emotions present at low intensity (perhaps especially interest and anxiety, but also anger, sadness, or shame) establish background feelings (Damasio, 1994) or moods (Davidson, 1994) that may not be observable in overt behavior, but still influence our thought and imagination, what we attend to and think about. Davidson has proposed that [whereas] "the primary function of emotion is to modulate and bias action . . . the primary function of moods . . . is to modulate and bias cognition" (p. 51).[4] Dix (1991) notes that "even mild affect initiates some change in outlook or inclination" (p. 5).

In normal development, the child constructs increasingly differentiated emotional appraisals and more flexible action tendencies. The child learns, for example, a more complex understanding of what makes him angry and different ways of being angry. In Izard's approach, emotion "recruits the cognitive system, rapidly and automatically," establishing a bond between perception, feeling, and action. These bonds have been referred to by Izard as "affective—cognitive structures" (Izard, 1991); by Tomkins as "scenes," "scripts," and values (and then, in even more complex forms, as ideology) (Demos, 1995); by Lewis and Douglas (1998) as "emotional interpretations"; and by Frijda, more simply, as "beliefs" (Frijda, 2007). In Izard's theory, affective—cognitive structures constitute "the most common type of mental structure . . . the fundamental building block of mind and memory." A feeling of joy linked with an image of a mother's face is a simple affective—cognitive structure; how a child imagines being comforted, or what a child imagines when she is angry, are more complex structures or beliefs.

With maturation and emotional development, both the expression and the experience of emotion are socialized and subject to complex transformations. Socializing influences, including cultural rules and practices (for example, that boys should not cry) modify the child's expression of emotion; an experienced emotion therefore will not, as in early childhood, invariably result in an observable response.[5] The socialization of emotional expression is a concern of parents in all cultures and a source of wide cultural variation in how and when emotions are expressed. In all cultures, children are taught—and observe—standards of behavior that include how and when to express emotions. Children are taught, for example, to inhibit, or regulate, expressions of anger and sadness; and socializing agents—parents and teachers—make increasing demands for mature or modulated expressions of emotion. Parents seek consultation with child clinicians when children frequently violate these expectations, when, for example, children continue to cry or have temper tantrums in response to minor frustrations and disappointments (or, less frequently, when children fail to express emotions that would be expected, especially in circumstances that normally evoke strong emotions).

Lewis and Douglas (1998) have presented a description of emotional development based on dynamic systems theory. In this approach, the child's emotional interpretations function as "attractors" in the child's "emotional landscape"—states of mind and patterns of behavior the child returns to with increasing frequency and which then become resistant to change.[6] In this way, emotional experiences become increasingly stable elements of a child's personality and character.

Because expressions of emotion include features that are invariant and universally recognizable (for example, typical facial expressions) as well as considerable individual and cultural variation, Fischer, Shaver, and Carnochan (1990) (see also Barrett and Campos, 1987) have proposed that different emotions are best understood as prototypes. The prototype of each emotion consists of "appraisals or appreciations, patterned physiological processes, action tendencies, subjective feelings, expressions, and instrumental behaviors" (p. 85). We are able to recognize an emotional experience—in ourselves and in others—as an instance of a particular emotion family based on its resemblance to the prototype, although none of the features of the prototype is invariably or necessarily present. Each emotion prototype has a "script" structure that specifies both typical antecedents and typical responses; for the negative emotions, the emotion script also includes self-control or coping strategies.

In the Fischer, Shaver, and Carnochan analysis, what "develops" in emotional development are emotional "skills"—more differentiated appraisals of emotionally-relevant events and more differentiated behavioral responses, that is, more flexible and adaptive emotion scripts. The child learns, for example, to understand and evaluate (appraise or appreciate) frustrations and disappointments—and her ability to cope with them—in a more differentiated way; every frustration or injury no longer evokes anger and blame. This critical development, which includes the child's increasing awareness of her emotions and the emotions of others, and the ability to regulate her emotional responses, has been described by Saarni (1997) as "emotional competence" and by Salovey and Mayer (1990; Mayer and Salovey, 1997) as "emotional intelligence."

To briefly review: Emotions are complex functional wholes, comprised of appraisals, subjective experience, and action dispositions. Every emotion serves an adaptive biological function. Emotions are signals to others and to ourselves—evoked by concerns—that rapidly organize thought and action toward more effective adaptation in response to events that have survival value. Emotions prepare us for action; the action tendencies inherent in the experience of an emotion may be expressed in overt behavior, but also as thoughts, attitudes, and fantasy. Emotional appraisals include an appraisal of the person's coping potential. And emotional maturity involves the development of increasingly flexible and adaptive emotion scripts or beliefs—more differentiated appraisals of events and more effective modes of emotional expression. From a functionalist perspective, distinctions between affect, cognition, and behavior are often arbitrary: thinking (especially appraisals) influences feeling, and feeling influences (organizes and directs) thought and action.

Each of these aspects of emotions has significant implications for our understanding of normal and pathological development in childhood and for the therapeutic process when helping troubled children and families.

Emotion, Need, and Self

Emotions, Panksepp and Burgdorf (2003) write, are "the currency of the mind/brain economy" and, in my view, the essential language of therapeutic communication with children. Like currency, however, the child's emotions (all emotions, but especially the "self-evaluative" emotions of shame and pride) reflect something of even deeper, more intrinsic, value. The quality and intensity of a child's emotions at any moment reflect the state of the child's needs and concerns, or, more broadly, the child's "self." The philosopher Martha Nussbaum (2001) has argued that human emotions are essentially "eudaimonistic," that is, evoked by and "about" events that are important to our "happiness" or "flourishing." Children—all of us—feel most deeply about events we perceive to affirm or threaten our deepest needs. Nussbaum argues that emotions are "forms of evaluative judgment that ascribe to certain things and persons outside a person's own control great importance for the person's own flourishing" (p. 22) and that all "emotions . . . involve judgments about important things, judgments in which . . . we acknowledge our neediness and incompleteness before parts of the world we do not completely control" (p. 19). When we talk with children about their emotions we are always talking about what is *important* to them—what they care about, what *matters* to them—their needs, plans, goals, "projects" (Nussbaum), or concerns. As child therapists, it is essential, when we speak with children, that we communicate, in some way—in our words and tone of voice—the *importance* of the child's feelings. (And we now know, from the research of John Gottman and his colleagues, that a dismissive or derogatory attitude by parents toward a child's emotions has significant deleterious effects on children's physiological and behavioral adjustment, Gottman, Hooven, and Katz, 1997; Gotttman, 1997.) In childhood, the child's most important concerns are her need to feel safe and to feel loved, and for the safety and well-being of those she loves; her need for recognition and affirmation; for acceptance and belonging; for competitive success; and her need for some form of self-esteem—to feel good about herself—and about others.

To illustrate the helpfulness of a functionalist approach to understanding the child's emotions, I will present a brief developmental and functional analysis of some representative emotions that are especially important—and I believe underappreciated—in clinical work with children.

Interest

Consider, first, the emotion of interest. Interest is activated by the appraisal of *novelty* or perceptual salience. Frijda (2007) suggests that interest may be our most basic emotion, an emotion that motivates our engagement with the world. Children become interested in objects or sensations that are colorful, moving, rhythmic, harmonious, or, more generally, beautiful. Infants show intense interest in their mother's face, especially her eyes (Schore, 1998) and young children are wide–eyed in their curiosity and interest in the lives of their parents. The probable adaptive function of interest is to alert us to potential resources in the environment (resources that enhance survival and reproductive success) and to provide the motivation to seek out those resources—to explore and investigate. The characteristic subjective experience associated with interest is *curiosity* or wonder (and, perhaps, "wanting," Panksepp, 1998, p. 245). The characteristic action dispositions associated with interest are search, exploration, and learning[7].

Izard and Ackerman (2000) remind us that interest "animates and enlivens the mind and body." Interest is "the mechanism of selective attention—the mechanism that keeps attention from straying more or less randomly through the vast array of stimuli that constantly impinge upon the senses." These authors cite Tomkins' view that "interest is the only emotion that can sustain long term constructive or creative endeavors" and report this somewhat surprising fact: "Healthy people in a safe and comfortable environment experience interest far more of the time than any other emotion" (p. 257).

Panksepp (1998) considers interest to be the characteristic affect of a basic emotional brain circuit he calls SEEKING. "These circuits appear to be major contributors to our feelings of engagement and excitement as we seek the material resources needed for bodily survival, and also when we pursue the cognitive interests that bring positive existential meaning to our lives" (p. 144). Activation of these circuits, whether normally occurring or artificially induced, fires "a positive, interest—filled engagement in the world" and more effective cortical processing; damage to this system results in a generalized behavioral inertia. When these neural systems are inactive (as in the cases of encephalitis-induced parkinsonism described by Oliver Sacks in *Awakenings*, 1973) "human aspirations remain frozen, as it were, in an endless winter of discontent." In contrast, when these "synapses are active in abundance, a person feels as if he/she can do anything." Panksepp suggests that "intense interest," "engaged curiosity," and "eager anticipation" are the characteristic subjective experiences associated with the arousal of these brain systems in humans (pp. 144–150).[8]

The importance of interest has also been noted by philosophers and artists. Bertrand Russell (1930) observed that, "young children are interested in everything that they see and hear." Russell regarded "zest"—a quality he defined as a person's interest in and enjoyment of many things—as "the most universal and distinctive mark of happy men" (p. 110). (Russell added that "genuine zest is part of the natural order of things" and "a feeling of being loved promotes zest more than anything else.") In the annotations that accompany his series of paintings, The Voyage of Life, the American landscape painter Thomas Cole wrote, "Joyousness and wonder are the characteristic emotions of childhood" (Powell, 1990).

Silvia (2005) has recently presented an experimental analysis of interest. In a series of studies, adult subjects were presented stimuli of different kinds and modalities: visual art, random polygons, and poetry. The subjects' degree of interest in these stimuli was determined by two factors: (1) the novelty of the stimulus presented and (2) the subject's appraisal of his or her ability to cope with new and complex things. For example, subjects spent more time viewing pictures and judged them as more interesting (although not more enjoyable) "when the picture was highly complex and they felt highly able to understand complex art" (p. 97).

In a slightly different formulation, based on my discussions with children about their varied interests, I would offer the hypothesis that, in everyday life, interest is *evoked* by the perception of novelty or beauty (e.g., by things that are colorful, sound harmonious, or move gracefully) and *sustained* by the expectation of eventual success; and that the experience of interest is enhanced, in childhood and throughout life, by *relevance*—that is, the extent to which we are able to perceive some relationship between this stimulus and other events. A sound or visual image (or a word, a movement, or an idea) is "interesting" to us to the extent (1) that it is novel; (2) that we feel competent to cope with the intellectual challenge (complexity) presented; and (3) that we are able to perceive some relationship between this sound or image (or idea) and other sounds or ideas, or to the solution of a practical concern. Children express interest—or lack of interest—in different activities for the same reasons. For the child who is interested in music (or in art, poetry, or athletics), the sound that she hears (or images, words, or movements) evoke other sounds, images, words, or movements and "light up" the child's brain.[9]

Interest is of critical importance in clinical work with children, in several respects. First, a therapist's (or parent's) enthusiastic responsiveness to a child's expressions of interest is the surest way to engage a child in some form of dialogue or interaction, and the surest way of conveying our desire to get to know a child. And it is through the sharing of interests that children begin to make friends. This is a first lesson of clinical work with children at any age: children respond to our animated expressions of *interest* in their *interests* with evident pleasure. In my clinical and supervisory experience, it is not unusual for children to express great pleasure when we respond to their interests in this way—they enjoy this form of interaction and want more of it. After even a brief period of responsive play, for example, a child may comment, "Mommy, this is fun. Can you sign me up for this?" or "Can I come here every day?" We offer, in this way, a kind of interaction that engages the child—and is often missing in the hurried, competitive, achievement-focused lives of many contemporary families.

Parents often express concern about the limited range of their child's interests or about their child's failure to sustain interest (and effort) toward important goals. We may be told, "She's not *interested* in reading (or writing, or drawing, or riding a bicycle). She's only interested in watching TV and playing video games." And many parents express frustration and dismay at their unsuccessful efforts to encourage, by any means—with any form of cajoling, rewards, or punishment—an expansion of the child's interests. As with all emotional and behavioral problems of childhood, the role of the child's temperament must be considered as a factor in determining the child's interests and in evaluating these complaints. In most instances, however, we may reasonably suspect that some pathologic process—anxiety, frustration, lack of confidence, or argument and protest—has restricted the range of the child's interests. The child's lack of interest and effort most often reflect an inarticulate feeling of frustration and perhaps also shame, and therefore avoidance. For the child who is not "interested" in reading or writing, it is likely that learning to read and write—the need to process the phonological structure of words, to formulate ideas, to recall and execute motor plans—does not come easily. The child's lack of *interest* in reading is the result of her *frustration* in learning to read; and her frustration is then expressed as avoidance and protest.

Finally, interest, like every emotion, evokes imagination and fantasy. In childhood, these may especially be fantasies of what the child is able to do or become, perhaps a policeman, an actor, or a poet. In the classical psychoanalytic theory, children are taught, or instinctively know, that some interests are forbidden, and the fantasies associated with these interests evoke anxiety and guilt.

Shame and Pride

The shame and pride family of emotions are core emotional experiences—in childhood and throughout life. Despite general recognition of the importance of chronic feelings of shame in adult psychopathology, the emotions of shame and pride receive insufficient attention—usually only passing mention—in most theories of emotional development in childhood.[10] As "self-conscious" or "self-evaluative" emotions, feelings of shame and pride more directly and immediately reflect the child's sense of self than other emotions, for example, anxiety, sadness, or anger. The child's need to mitigate feelings of shame—and to maintain or restore a feeling of pride—is a fundamental motivational principle and an essential constituent of emotional health.

Shame is evoked, throughout life, by personal failure or inadequacy, especially the public exposure of inadequacy. In childhood, adolescence, and in adult life, the shame family of emotions includes a range of subjective experiences, from mild embarrassment to deeply painful feelings of humiliation, aloneness, and self-hatred. Izard (1991) cites Darwin's opinion that shame is most often evoked by "blame, criticism and derision" (p. 338). Children experience feelings of shame when they suffer social rejection; when they are unable to learn; when they are defeated in any competitive encounter; when they are bullied, insulted (Gilligan, 2003), or taunted; and when they seek acceptance and approval from admired adults but are, instead, subject to criticism or "derogation" (Gottman, Hooven, and Katz, 1997). Many experiences that evoke a feeling of shame—for example, experiences of exclusion or ridicule—are uniquely painful, and the feeling of shame is difficult to get rid of.

The characteristic subjective experience of shame is a feeling of being exposed, inferior or unworthy, of shrinking, and of heightened self-consciousness (Barrett, 1995; Izard, 1991).[11] The characteristic action disposition associated with the emotion of shame is *concealment*; we all attempt to hide or cover up what we are ashamed of. Pride is antithetical to shame. The characteristic action tendency associated with pride is an *outward* movement and the inclination to show and tell others, to exhibit or "show off." Pride is *expansive*, in both action and imagination; shame *contracts*, in posture, and also in thought and imagination—in the setting of goals and in what the child considers possible for herself.[12]

H. B. Lewis (1971; 1989), in an influential phenomenological analysis of shame and guilt, notes that shame is evoked by the experience of failure—sexual failure, failure in competition, moral failure or transgression—and by social rejection. Lewis suggests that we feel *guilt* "about *things* done or not done in the world;" *shame*, in contrast, involves "the whole *self*. It is the vicarious experience of the other's scorn of the self" (1989, p. 40). Lewis offers the general formulation that, "both shame and guilt are affective-cognitive signals that the attachment system is threatened, and both states push the individual toward repairing and restoring affectional bonds." (p. 36). Some, although not all, experiences of shame also evoke a distinct and intense form of retaliatory anger that Lewis calls *humiliated fury* and that Kohut (1972) described as narcissistic rage.[13]

In a somewhat different analysis, Weisfeld (1997) has argued, from an evolutionary perspective, that the emotions of shame and pride represent opposite poles of a single emotion system, derived from instinctive expressions of social status. Weisfeld suggests that the postural and vocal expressions of shame originated as signals of submission in competitive encounters, thereby saving the life of the loser by protecting him from further aggression and eliciting communal support. Competitive defeat (and perhaps also social exclusion) may therefore be the prototypic experience of shame; competitive victory may be the prototypic experience of pride.

Following Darwin, Weisfeld notes that "pride and shame have distinct, stereotypic expressions" (p. 428): "Proud, successful people carry themselves expansively and conspicuously; their gaze is direct, especially while speaking, and their manner is relaxed. And they want people to look at them." In this analysis, the experience of pride evolved from expressions of *dominance* and still involves displays of dominance. The unabashed triumphant bragging of young boys and the more (or less) socialized exhibitionistic displays of victorious adult males (and the bragging of parents and grandparents about the accomplishments of their offspring) are instinctive expressions of pride.

Gilbert (2003; Gilbert and McGuire, 1998) offers a similar evolutionary theory of the origins of shame. Gilbert suggests that the experiences of pride and shame originated in ongoing evaluations of our relative fighting ability, and now continue as we monitor our social attractiveness—our ability to elicit approval and acceptance, to obtain recognition, and to be desirable to others. In this instinctive competition "to be liked, approved of, and valued," shame is a signal that we have failed. The feeling of shame therefore functions as "...an inner warning signal of threats and challenges to the self" (Gilbert, 2003, p. 1205).[14] Although there are unresolved differences in these various understandings of shame, Weisfeld is undoubtedly correct when he asserts that, "We anticipate pride and shame at every turn and shape our behavior accordingly" (p. 426).

Shame may have additional, important social functions. Because shame is evoked by the anticipation of scorn or disapproval, Izard (1991) suggests that the experience of shame may function to promote conformity and social cohesion, including the recognition of authority and superior status, and acceptance of community standards. Izard argues that, "Avoidance of shame can thus be seen as a powerful motive for social conformity and individual responsibility" (p. 341).

J. Gilligan (2003), based on extensive interviews with violent criminals, has argued that "the basic psychological motive, or cause, of violent behavior is the wish to ward off or eliminate the feeling of shame and humiliation...and replace it with its opposite, the feeling of pride" (p. 1154). Gilligan believes that shame "is the pathogen that causes violence just as specifically as the tubercle bacillus causes tuberculosis, except that in the case of violence it is an emotion, not a microbe" (p. 1155).

M. Lewis (2003) reports that behavioral and postural expressions typical of the experience of shame—bodily collapse, shoulders falling in, gaze downward or askance—can be reliably observed in 3-year-olds by exposing the child to experimentally induced "failure" at simple tasks. J. Kagan (1984) reports a likely precursor to the emotion of shame in the observation that 2-year-old children from diverse cultures will protest and cry when they are unable to repeat a sequence of actions they have just observed. Schore (1998) suggests that children experience shame even earlier, in the second year of life, as a response to expressions of disapproval, or when the child is unable to elicit joyful affect (e.g., a smile) in face-to-face interactions with caregivers. Children with difficulties in motor coordination or delays in language development that impede the development of physical or language competence may experience a form of shame early in childhood; somewhat later, difficulties in learning, especially in learning to read, evoke a profound feeling of shame. Empathic adults (and often other children), even empathic chimpanzees, recognize this emotional state and instinctively offer consolations (DeWaal, 2001), in an effort to mitigate the child's feeling of shame.

There is also some controversy about the emergence of pride. Children are observed, as early as age 18 months, to smile after completing a task; Kagan (1984) refers to these as "mastery smiles." Even earlier, infants show joy and delight "as the result of having some effect on the environment or... exercising some emerging skill" (Stipek, 1995, p. 237). It is likely that these experiences of success, or "making things happen," represent a precursor or an early form of pride. Most developmental theorists, however, distinguish this delight from pride on the basis that pride requires evidence of a self-conscious or self-reflective evaluation. Unambiguous expressions of pride (for example, smiling *and* turning to look at an adult following the successful completion of a task) are observed between 2 and 3 years old (Stipek, 1995).

The child's anticipation of feeling proud or feeling ashamed plays a critical role in her emotional and behavioral adjustment. These self-evaluative processes—what children feel they are "good at" and "not good at"; whether they are liked or disliked, admired or scorned—are continually present, throughout childhood and throughout life, experienced as an essential aspect of our conscious sense of self-esteem, or as "implicit self attitudes" (Conner and Barrett, 2005). The child's expectation of feeling proud or ashamed decisively influences her choices—those situations she actively seeks or avoids—and her ability to sustain effort toward goals. Weisfeld notes that shame (our emotional response to failure) lowers aspirations; pride (an outcome of success) "raises aspirations" (p. 432). When children are anxious, they are often anxious about the possibility of feeling ashamed. Prolonged feelings of shame are profoundly pathogenic, leading to avoidance, depression, and withdrawal, and, increasingly in adolescence, to desperate attempts to alleviate—or get rid of—this painful state of mind.

The need to maintain, or restore, a feeling of pride is essential to mental health and remains a fundamental human motivation throughout the life span, both in our private as well as in our public, political lives. In childhood and throughout life, we need to celebrate our accomplishments (and, perhaps, to feel superior to someone else). Experiences that mitigate feelings of shame and restore a feeling of pride—experiences that confer status, respect, being looked up to, being "the best at"—become highly valued, core aspects of our character and behavior.

Anxiety

Anxiety is perhaps the most extensively studied emotion, especially its pathological manifestations as worry, phobia, or obsession. Individual differences in "anxiety sensitivity" (Reiss, Silverman, and Weems, 2001) and behavioral inhibition (Biederman et al., 1993), biological risk factors for the development of anxiety disorders in childhood and adolescence, have been reliably established;

and effective cognitive-behavioral treatments for some childhood anxiety disorders have been developed (Kendall, Aschenbrand, and Hudson, 2003).

Anxiety is evoked by the anticipation of physical or psychological danger and "uncertainty about the ability to control outcomes" (Chorpita, 2001). Ohman (2000) explains that "the responses of fear and anxiety originate in an alarm system shaped by evolution to protect creatures from impending danger" (p. 587). Following a distinction proposed by Epstein, Ohman suggests that *fear* motivates escape or avoidance; we become *anxious* about events we are afraid of, but that we cannot escape or avoid (e.g., an examination).[15]

In its most adaptive function, anxiety motivates caution and preparedness. The principal cognitive manifestation of anxiety is "increased stimulus analysis" (Chorpita, 2001), a cognitive bias to attend to possible threat, and a narrowing of the focus of attention to the source of threat. The principal behavioral response associated with anxiety is seeking safety and security, evident, for example, in the proximity-seeking behavior of young children and, throughout life, in more complex forms of proximity-seeking and avoidance of danger (including various forms of cognitive disengagement, for example, repression, selective inattention, and dissociation). Our experience of anxiety, perhaps more obviously than any other emotion, depends on an appraisal of our coping potential—whether we feel able to cope with the threat or challenge presented.

Like interest, anxiety is almost continually present, or easily evoked, as a background factor or mood; at the very least, anxiety is a daily experience in the lives of children, as they anticipate interactions with parents, teachers, and peers. Izard (1991) recalls Lorenz's instructive example of the reciprocal relationship of interest and anxiety. Lorenz watched a raven, perched a high limb of a tall tree, cautiously approach an object on the ground. The raven flew towards the object of interest and would then retreat to the safety of successively lower branches. Children, like Lorenz's raven, are interested, but also anxious, in their anticipation of any novel situation, for example, their first day of school or summer camp. They are anxious in anticipation of criticism and punishment; about separation, loss, and pain; and about their first encounter with a child therapist. They are perhaps especially anxious about experiences that may evoke feelings of shame (for example, social rejection, academic failure, or an evaluation or performance of any kind). Attentive parents recognize this emotional state and, in myriad ways, but especially with their presence and encouragement, help the child learn to "cope" with her anxiety, keeping anxiety within a tolerable range, so that the child can explore, then safely retreat, then explore again. The child then learns to approach new situations with greater interest (as an opportunity) and less fear.[16]

Anger

Anger, as is well known, is evoked by frustration (i.e., interference with obtaining desired goals; not getting what we want or deserve), by feeling "wronged" (Miller and Sperry, 1987),[17] and by physical or emotional pain and injury. In my view, the pathogenic role of persistent anger—in the form of resentment and grievance, defiance, and withdrawal—remains insufficiently appreciated in many current theories of pathological development in childhood.

Although still subject to some controversy, expressions of anger can first be reliably observed in infancy at 3 or 4 months of age, in response to arm restraint or inoculations (Lemerise and Dodge, 2000); and throughout life, restraint on our freedom of movement (or restrictions on any of our freedoms) remains a significant source of anger. Panksepp (1998) presents the intriguing hypothesis that vigorous movement in response to physical restraint, an effective means by which captured prey are able to escape from the grasp of predators, may have been the evolutionary origin of anger in mammals.[18] As adults, as in childhood, we become angry when we are injured or held back, and at any potential harm to people or things we love or value. The contemporary adaptive function of anger, broadly defined, is therefore to defend ourselves and those we love. In families, children become angry in response to emotional injuries (especially criticism and exclusion) and when the resources they value—whether these are material "things" or, more importantly, recognition and approval—are allocated unfairly.

The characteristic action disposition of anger is some form of protest or attack—an effort to remove the source of frustration or pain. Miller and Sperry offer this concise definition: "Anger is the felt need to retaliate" (p. 5). Again, this action tendency may be expressed in behavior or in imagination. When children have been hurt, their thought and imagination are recruited into the service of justifying retaliation, especially by blaming—"our mental dialogues overflow with statements of blame and scorn" (Panksepp, 1998, p. 191). Because emotions bias perception, anger that remains active is likely to find expression in a readiness to perceive potential threats—any movement (or spoken word), for example, is more likely to be interpreted as a possible provocation or attack. The form and intensity of a child's protest or retaliation is, of course, highly variable, depending on the child's character and personality; on the context, both past and present, of the child's frustration or injury; on the maturation of the child's capacity for expression of emotion; and on how the expression of anger has been socialized. With development, appraisals of intentionality play an increasingly important role in the child's experience of anger. Anger is evoked (or, perhaps, justified) by appraisals that the frustration or injury was intentional or "unfair." (For this reason, parents often attempt to calm an angry child by explaining, "He didn't mean it" or "It was just an accident.")

Developmental research on anger (see Lemerise and Dodge, 2000, for a review) has focused on anger that is evoked by frustration—an obstruction or interference with the child's plans or goals. Conclusions derived from this research are important and not surprising: Children who are able to regulate their expressions of anger are better liked by their peers, as early as preschool, and a child's inability to regulate expressions of anger is an established risk factor for psychopathology at all ages. When parents are often angry at their children, children show increased "distress, avoidant interaction styles, less prosocial behavior toward parents and peers, and poorer understanding of emotion" (p. 598).

Because of its obvious destructive potential, anger is, arguably, subject to earlier and greater socializing efforts than any other emotion. Children are explicitly taught when and how, under what circumstances and against whom, they are allowed to express anger, beginning in early childhood. (Preschool children, for example, are told, when they are angry, not to hit but, instead, to "use your words.") With development and increasing emotional maturity, children are expected to inhibit expressions of anger (especially toward teachers) and to express anger in planful (versus impulsive or urgent) ways.

Intense, often violent, anger is also evoked, in childhood and throughout life, in response to emotional injury. Kohut (1972) offered a brilliant description of this phenomenon in his concept of narcissistic rage, a qualitatively distinct form of anger evoked by narcissistic injury, and characterized, in its most extreme form, by an insatiable search for revenge. Narcissistic rage, perhaps more than restrictions on our freedoms, has played a profound—and profoundly destructive—role in human history. The historian Donald Kagan (1995), in his studies of the origins of war, notes, "how small a role... considerations of practical utility and material gain, and even ambition for power itself, play in bringing on wars, and how often some aspect of honor is decisive" (p. 8).

Successful programs have been developed to help children develop improved "anger management" (Lochman et al., 2006). These therapeutic interventions help children reevaluate events that elicit anger and generate alternative, less destructive methods of expressing anger. (See also Greenberg, 2006, for a discussion of the PATHS curriculum for reducing aggressive behavior through the development of improved executive functions in children.) In my view, we may be even more helpful if we define our clinical task more broadly: to identify the sources of the child's frustration and anger and, especially, to promote processes in families that repair feelings of resentment and grievance. We would then not only help children "manage" their anger; they would be less angry in the first place.

Sadness

Sadness is our instinctive response to loss, aloneness (whether physical or psychological aloneness), and disappointment. We experience sadness especially at the loss of someone (or something) we deeply value and at the loss of sources of affirmation and support—the loss of those who have helped us thrive. The probable origin and adaptive function of expressions of sadness in mammals is to elicit social support (especially in the form of physical touch) when children have been separated from their parents (Panksepp, 1998). Prolonged sadness (grief), characterized by behavioral withdrawal and the slowing of psychological and physical systems, may have evolved to serve the conservation of resources when distress calls do not elicit an immediate response, and perhaps also to allow recuperation from injury and infection (Maier and Watkins, 1998). In modern human life, sadness has come to serve a more general adaptive function: We are motivated by sadness, and learn from sadness, to appreciate, protect, and preserve what we value.[19] Perhaps for this reason, in some cultures and historical eras (including, to some extent, our own) the experience of sadness has been regarded as a virtue, derived from an appreciation of the tragic dimension of life, and associated with patience, maturity, and wisdom (as, for example, in Coleridge's famous poem, "The Rime of the Ancient Mariner": "A sadder and a wiser man/he woke the morrow morn.") Most, if not all, human societies have constructed rituals and belief systems that serve, at least in part, this function: to mitigate our experience of sadness and loss, and to preserve the memory of those we have loved.

Sadness and disappointment, however, are also common, perhaps daily, events in the life of the child. Children experience sadness in reaction to ordinary disappointments as well as profound sadness in response to extraordinary, traumatic events (for example, prolonged separation, divorce, or death). In these moments, empathic parents offer solace and consolation to the child, and help the child learn that this disappointment, although sad, will not last forever. In this way, the child develops the ability to *tolerate* disappointment, an essential component of emotional resilience. In contrast, prolonged sadness will bias the child's thinking toward the anticipation or expectation of future disappointments.

In Bowlby's (1980) theory, the original adaptive function and action tendency of sadness ("the cry of sorrow... tends to preserve the life of the young by bringing them who watch over them to their assistance," Shand, cited in Bowlby, p. 27) continues in human psychology as "a mourner is repeatedly seized, whether he knows it or not, by an urge to call for, to search for and to recover the lost person." Bowlby cites examples of how very young children unconsciously attempt to preserve the memory of an absent parent. For example, one child, Philip, placed in a residential nursery at age 13 months, would "make the motions associated with the rhyme... his mother used to humor him" (p. 11).

The child's efforts to cope with loss and preserve loved people and objects are beautifully illustrated in two of my favorite books for children. *Geraldine's Blanket*, by Holly Keller (1984), describes a young child's attachment to a "security" blanket. "Geraldine," the book begins, "had a pink blanket. Aunt Bessie sent it when Geraldine was a little baby. Geraldine took it everywhere with her." The blanket becomes worn and frayed, but Geraldine rebuffs all her parents' efforts to convince her to give up her blanket. The parents then try a different approach. A new present arrives from

Aunt Bessie—a wonderful doll named Rosa. Geraldine loves the new doll, but she still will not give up her blanket. Then Geraldine has an idea—she takes the now tattered blanket and makes it into a coat for Rosa. She says, "Now Rosa has the blanket and I have Rosa." This brief story illustrates an important psychological process in coping with sadness. Faced with the loss of a loved and sustaining object, Geraldine finds a *generative* solution to her problem. She can now experience herself as both solacing as well as solaced (Adams-Silvan and Silvan, 1988) and she can feel sustained by her own caring activity.

In *My Grandmother's Cookie Jar*, by Montzalee Miller (1987), a young Native American girl listens to the stories her grandmother lovingly tells her every night about "her Indian people of long ago," as they eat cookies together from a special jar. When the grandmother dies, the girl's grandfather consoles her. He brings her the empty cookie jar and gently explains, "The jar is full of Grandma's love and Indian spirit. When you are grown and have children of your own you will put cookies in the jar. The cookies will be dusted with Grandma's love. If you tell one of grandma's stories with each of the cookies, then her spirit and the spirit of those who went before her will live on." The young girl resolves, "I will keep the spirits alive. I will tell grandmother's stories."

Most of us can probably recall, in our own lives, moments of sadness or loneliness, followed, when we are fortunate, as in Miller's moving story, by a resolve—to make this sadness meaningful by creating a more meaningful life. Such moments, in varying degrees of intensity, are perhaps a universal accompaniment to the process of separation and individuation that normally occurs in adolescence and early adulthood. How we resolve these crises of sadness comes to define, in large part, our character and guiding values.

Notes

1. See, for example, Barrett, 1995; 1998; Barrett and Campos, 1987; Fischer, Shaver, and Carnochan, 1990; Fischer and Tangney, 1995; Griffin and Mascolo, 1998; Gross and Thompson, 2007; Izard, 1991; and Nussbaum, 2001. Gross and Thompson refer to this emerging consensus as a "modal" model of emotions. See also Panksepp, 1998, for a discussion of ongoing controversies.
2. Dix (1991) offers the following concise explanation of a functionalist understanding of emotion: "Once activated, emotions transform people's orientation toward the environment... emotions activate, orient, and organize adaptive processes. They are characterized by changes in cognition, physiology, motivation, subjective feeling states, behavioral readiness, and facial and vocal expressions. These changes prepare people to perceive and evaluate particular features of events (cognition), activate motives to seek out particular outcomes (motivation), communicate to others the person's affective stance (expressive behavior), and prepare response tendencies likely to be needed (behavioral inclinations)" (p. 5).

3. "Affects... signal the survival value of objects and ways of acting in the world" (Panksepp and Burgdorf, 2003) and "alert the organism to the need for further information processing and action" (Clark and Watson, 1994, p. 131). Panksepp (2007) notes that "affect encodes for value" and these values establish "comfort zones by which animals, including humans, live their lives."
4. "Mood serves as a primary mechanism for altering information-processing priorities and for shifting modes of information processing. Mood will accentuate the accessibility of some and attenuate the accessibility of other cognitive contents and semantic networks. For example, individuals in a depressed mood have increased accessibility to sad memories and decreased accessibility to happy memories" (Davidson, 1994, p. 52).
5. Izard and Ackerman explain: "In infants, the processes that activate an emotion typically lead to some expressive behavior. As a function of both maturation and socialization, however, the relations between neural activation processes and expressive behavior change... Eventually, observable expression in some situations may be completely inhibited or disassociated." Izard and Ackerman also note that, "A child learning to regulate emotion *expressions* is part of the process of learning to regulate emotion *experiences*" (p. 256).
6. "When particular ways of seeing the world recur over occasions, attractors become deeper and more specific, constituting developmental change" (p. 170). See also Granic and Patterson (2006), for a dynamic systems theory analysis of antisocial development, discussed in Chapter 3.
7. It is possible that our appreciation of beauty in a more general sense—a universal human characteristic—evolved from this basic emotional response.
8. What Panksepp relabels SEEKING circuits were called, in classic neuroscience studies, "reward" or "pleasure" centers, because laboratory animals would work, often to exhaustion, for the opportunity to provide self-stimulation to these brain regions. Panksepp argues, however, that this is not a reward or reinforcement system, but a basic neurological system for exploration. He notes that "people [who have had artificial stimulation of these brain regions] typically report not simple sensory pleasures, but rather, invigorated feelings that are difficult to describe. They commonly report a feeling that something very interesting and exciting is going on" (p. 149).
9. Cf. Gardner's (1983) discussion of multiple intelligences in *Frames of Mind*.
10. For a well-known exception, see Erikson, 1950.
11. Shame and pride, like all emotions, are also associated with characteristic vocal patterns and complex physiological reactions (Barrett, 1995).
12. Izard, however, in what appears to be a minority view, does not regard pride as a discrete emotion. Instead, Izard considers pride (like envy, jealousy, or humility) a complex affective-cognitive structure or "state of mind."
13. Lewis also offers the important clinical insight that unacknowledged shame in the patient –therapist relationship is a common cause of treatment failure.
14. Scheff (1998) cites Cooley's analysis that "pride and shame serve as intense and automatic bodily signs of the state of a system that is difficult to observe. Pride is the sign of an intact social bond; shame is the sign of a threatened one.... Pride and shame thus serve as instinctive signals, both to the self and to the other, that communicate the state of that bond" (p. 192).

15. Freud (1926), in his revision of the psychoanalytic theory of anxiety, posited a developmental sequence of anxiety or danger situations in childhood, beginning with the child's fear of loss of the object, and continuing with fear of loss of the object's love, fear of punishment (castration), and finally, fear of conscience.
16. Current therapeutic approaches to anxiety in children (Kendall and Suveg, 2006) attempt to mitigate one or more components of the anxiety response: (1) through cognitive reappraisals of the danger situation, i.e., the child's imaginings of the likelihood of danger; (2) by reducing the physiological arousal associated with anxiety; and/or (3) by strengthening the child's confidence in her capacity to cope with the challenge presented. Research is now focused on the question of whether different subgroups of anxious children respond differentially to one of these components of therapeutic interventions (Eisen and Silverman, 1993, 1998, cited in Ollendick, King, and Chorpita, 2006).
17. Miller and Sperry (1987): "Anger and aggression... originate... in a person's perception that he or she has been thwarted or wronged" (p. 5).
18. On several occasions, I have been consulted by parents who had been advised to "hold" (physically restrain) their angry children. This recommendation is based on what I believe is a perverse concretization of Winnicott's concept of a child's need for "holding." Although, in some cases, the technique of "holding" may seem to "work" (that is, the child becomes calmer), it is likely that the child has simply given up in her struggle against a stronger adversary; her anger, however, has been significantly intensified and will likely find some other form of expression—in fantasy or in future acts of defiance and aggression.
19. Sadness serves to "help people become more aware of... [and] conserve what is important, and more particularly to maintain attachment to others" (Barr-Zisowitz, 2000, p. 618).

2

Optimal and Pathological Development in Childhood: A General Theory

Optimal Development: Resilience and Positive Expectations

Drawing on this understanding of the nature of emotions and emotional development, I would now like to propose an emotion-based theory of optimal and pathological development in childhood. In this model, the psychopathology of childhood and adolescence, whether expressed as a disturbance of mood or behavior, results from the persistence of negative emotions—and the complex transformations of these emotions—in the mind of the child.

Psychological health, from this perspective, is characterized by a predominance of *positive* emotions and positive *expectations*—an expansion of thoughts and fantasies (or scripts or beliefs) associated with the affects of interest, excitement, joy, pride, and love. In optimal development, the child's experience is characterized by a mood or background feeling of *interest* and the *expectation* of pleasurable and affirming interactions. In health, children are able to express a range of emotion (Emde, 1991) and the child will more often look forward to (appraise or appreciate) events in his life as situations of interest and opportunity, rather than anxiety or threat. Emotional health also involves some degree of optimism (cf. Seligman, 1995), a child's hopeful sense of his future. In these optimal circumstances, the child's behavior will predominantly be guided by his anticipation and active seeking of affirming experiences and positive emotions, rather than seeking escape or relief from painful emotions.[1]

Optimal development is also characterized by a second, decisive factor. In psychological health, children learn that emotional distress is temporary; that through their own actions, or with the help of supportive adults, they can make things better—that they need not remain anxious, sad, or angry. In this way, the child develops the capacity to *tolerate* negative emotions and to quickly recover, or bounce back, from the inevitable disappointments and frustrations of childhood. This capacity will be manifest as *emotional resilience,* or what Horton and Gewirtz (1988) refer to as "psychological immunity." The development of emotional resilience—the child's ability to restore, following disappointments and emotional injuries, some good feeling about himself and others and some form of positive expectation—is, in my view, the critical variable in the psychological health of the child and the central goal of our therapeutic efforts.

In these optimal circumstances, when children are able to bounce back from frustration and disappointment, maturing processes and pro-social development take place. The child develops a more differentiated appraisal of events and more adaptive modes of coping with the expectable stresses of daily life. The child who is more able to tolerate distress will be more successful in his peer relationships (Gottman, Katz, and Hooven, 1997), more willing to compromise, to take into account the needs of others, and more open to the socializing efforts of parents and educators.

In contrast, pathological development is characterized by an elaboration or strengthening, in the mind and behavior of the child, of thoughts and action tendencies associated with painful affects. Painful emotions *remain active* in the mind of the child. The child's thought and imagination are increasingly absorbed in attitudes or fantasies associated with negative emotions and the development of scripts or beliefs (especially beliefs about himself) dominated by anger, shame, anxiety, and sadness.

In pathological development, the child's emotional life is characterized by qualities of *urgency* and *inflexibility*.[2] The child's thinking becomes increasingly *vigilant* and less open—focused on anticipating and avoiding threats, rather than finding possibilities—often, with a consequent restriction in the range of the child's interests and imaginative development. Thoughts and expectations associated with painful affects become strengthened; the physiological arousal associated with painful emotions also remains present or is more easily activated; and the child's behavior is characterized by increasing defiance or withdrawal. A child's failure to tolerate, or bounce back, from painful affects will often be manifest in persistent and urgent protests and demands, or persistent avoidance and withdrawal. These maladaptive strategies for coping with painful affects will also, in almost every instance, result in some failure in the development of successful socialization and peer relationships.

From this perspective, the measure of pathological development in childhood is the degree to which negative affects—and the thoughts and behavioral tendencies associated with these emotions—have come to dominate the mind of the child. In pathology, the experience of painful affects, especially shame and anger, has become habitual and pervasive, and has increasingly shaped the development of the child's moods and behavior, of personality and character, and of parent-child and peer relationships. Severe emotional and behavioral pathology in childhood and adolescence (and in many adults as well) results from painful affects that the child cannot "get rid of" and therefore continue to influence his sense of himself and others.

In healthy development, children learn, with increasing sophistication, to modulate both their experience and their expression of negative affects.

This important development is frequently discussed as the capacity for affect or emotion regulation. Emotion dysregulation is now recognized as a critical general factor in the development of many forms of child psychopathology, both internalizing and externalizing disorders (Bradley, 2000; Cole and Zahn-Waxler, 1992; Fonagy et al., 2002; Keenan, 2000; Schore, 1994; Tyson, 1998). More fundamentally, in my opinion, children learn not merely to *regulate* their emotions; they learn that painful feelings are *temporary* and therefore bearable—not catastrophic and not forever. In this way, the child learns to *tolerate* painful emotions.

Consider, again, a child's feeling of shame. In pathological development, shame *remains active* in the mind of the child. Persistent, or easily evoked, feelings of shame will be expressed in the child's conscious or unconscious self-evaluation as in some way inferior or unworthy; in his expectation of conspicuous failure or defeat; and in a readiness to perceive slights, or to feel exposed. Shame persists in thought as pessimism or feelings of inferiority and in behavior as avoidance or withdrawal—an avoidance of situations in which failure or disapproval is likely, or even possible. Persistent shame is also likely to intensify the child's feelings of envy. The child will more often feel, for example, "I wish I was as good as. . . ." or "as attractive as . . ." And, as J. Gilligan (2003) has proposed, the need to eradicate a sense of shame (and restore a feeling of pride and dignity) may be a cause of violence.

Anger that remains active will be expressed as some form of ongoing protest or argument; as a readiness—in fantasy or in action—to defy or disparage; and as attitudes of resentment and contempt. Chronic frustration, anger, and emotional pain lead all of us to harbor darker thoughts about others and about ourselves. A child who remains angry may begin to hold onto grievances, to inwardly "build a case" against offending others, to divide the world into "all good" and "all bad" (Kernberg, 1983), "enemies and allies" (Volkan, 1988), and to develop an intractable sense of unfairness and injustice. These children may also be more likely show the cognitive biases associated with aggressive behavior—vigilance, misattributions of hostile intent, and positive evaluation of aggressive strategies for solving interpersonal problems (Dodge, Bates, and Petit, 1990).

The child's clinical presentation—and our therapeutic task—is then complicated by the child's defenses—the child is increasingly engaged in some effort to hide, or get rid of, bad feelings. Painful affects will often be masked by denial and blaming, and the child comes to rely on dysfunctional modes of reducing distress—demands or avoidances, dissociative strategies, or attitudes of superiority and contempt.

This understanding of optimal and pathological development suggests a revised framework and goals for child psychotherapy. Our efforts in all phases of the therapeutic process will be directed toward the development of increased emotional resilience and psychological immunity—to promote processes in children and families that strengthen the child's positive expectations and mitigate the pathogenic influence of persistent negative emotions.

This salutary development will be manifest in the child's increased tolerance for painful affects, in less urgent and inflexible demands, in less frequent avoidance and withdrawal, and in more successful peer relationships—a more confident and joyful participation in life.[3]

How Does Emotional Resilience Develop?

But how does emotional resilience or psychological immunity develop? How do children develop the ability to tolerate negative emotions and bounce back from emotional distress? And how can we, in clinical work with children and families, promote resilience? The remainder of this book presents a multi-faceted answer to these fundamental questions. I will begin, in this chapter, with a brief review of some essential clinical theory and research: attachment theory, interactive repair processes, Heinz Kohut's developmental theory, and lessons learned from longitudinal studies of high-risk children.

Attachment and Interactive Repair

Over the past two decades, attachment theory has emerged as a compelling theoretical and research paradigm for the study of optimal and pathological development in childhood. This research has established basic principles, now widely accepted: (1) that attachment, or proximity-seeking, behaviors of children (and care-giving behaviors of parents) constitute a biologically adaptive behavioral system, activated in situations of danger, threat, or challenge; (2) that the availability and responsiveness of attachment figures serve an essential security and stress-regulatory function for the child; (3) that patterns of attachment behavior become prototypes for the child's subsequent affect-regulation strategies; (4) that experiences of parental responsiveness to the child's distress shape the child's expectations or representations of self and others (Slade, 1999; Sroufe et al., 2005); and (5) that secure or insecure attachment patterns establish an early developmental trajectory, influenced by subsequent events, that become risk or protective factors in the psychological development of the child. In optimal development, parental responsiveness to the child's distress establishes an expectation, or internal working model, of the availability of relief (or "re-equilibration," Fonagy and Target, 1998). This expectation reduces the child's arousal and allows the young child to explore his environment with greater confidence and freedom.

These ideas have received increasing empirical support (for a review, see Kobak et al., 2006; also Sroufe et al., 1999 and Sroufe et al., 2005). Many of the therapeutic recommendations I will present in later chapters, especially recommendations for parent guidance, serve to restore or strengthen a child's confident expectation of parental availability and emotional support, and are therefore consistent with these basic tenets of attachment theory.

The direct application of attachment theory to psychotherapy with school-age children, however, has been problematic. Most therapeutic programs for children based on attachment theory have been designed for very young children or children who have suffered traumatic life events (Oppenheim and Goldsmith, 2007).

In daily clinical practice with school-age children, a child's attachment status is not directly observable, and it is difficult (except in extreme cases—cases, for example, of abuse, neglect, or frequent disruptions of attachment) to obtain an independent assessment of a child's attachment history. As a result, although the child's capacity for affect regulation under conditions of stress, hypothesized as an outcome of secure attachment, is of central therapeutic importance, the etiological role of a child's attachment history remains speculative. In my own work, therefore, attachment theory does not often directly influence my clinical assessment of the child or of parent-child relationships. A related research program, however—the paradigm of interactive repair—offers a theory of resilience that has significant implications for therapeutic work with parents and children at all ages.

Interactive repair has been extensively studied by Tronick (1989; 2006). In FFSF (Face-to-Face Still-Face) research, mothers are instructed, following an episode of normal face-to-face social interaction, "to keep an unresponsive poker face and not smile, touch, or talk to the baby." Under these conditions, infants demonstrate what has been called the "still-face effect"—decreased positive affect, increased negative affect and gaze aversion, increased visual scanning and pick-me-up gestures, and, in more recent studies, evidence of increased physiological stress. When mothers resume normal interaction, infants return to a positive affective state and show a reduction of stress.

In a recent review of two decades of research, Tronick (2006) proposed a "normal stress-resilience hypothesis" of the development of resilience in infancy and early childhood. Tronick argues that the FFSF experimental paradigm provides "a model for *normal* interactions and the stress that accompanies them" (2006, p. 93) and that "behavioral and physiological resilience develops in part from infants' and young children's experience coping with the inherent normal stress of daily life and social interaction" (p. 94). Tronick suggests that children learn from repeated experiences of interactive repair, beginning in infancy, both that emotional distress is temporary (and therefore bearable) and that their own actions can bring about relief. In this way, "the infant develops a representation of himself or herself as effective, and of his or her interactions as positive and reparable" (pp. 94–95).[4]

It seems likely, as Tronick has proposed, that repeated experiences of interactive repair (or, more generally, recovery from distress) establish in the very young child a baseline of the child's capacity to regulate and bounce back from negative affect. It would be a mistake, however, to limit our understanding of this development to the early years of life. Throughout childhood, supportive parents continually try to keep their children's experience of anxiety and disappointment within "tolerable" limits and they offer myriad forms of emotional support that enable children to bear painful feelings; perhaps particularly important are the parents' capacity to provide empathy and solace (Horton and Gerwitz, 1988), to encourage the verbalization of affect states (Hooven, Gottman, and Katz, 1995; Katan, 1961) and ongoing parental expressions of pride, encouragement, and confidence in the child's and adolescent's mastery of developmental challenges. These experiences of emotional support—or the absence of emotional support—are often immediately accessible in daily clinical observations and offer important opportunities for therapeutic interventions.

Affirmation

Among the many theories of psychological development that have been presented, Heinz Kohut's proposals regarding the development of healthy narcissism and a "cohesive self" are especially relevant to the question of emotional resilience. Kohut's theory, highly influential over several decades in psychoanalysis, has received surprisingly little attention in child development research and child therapy, even among psychoanalytic child therapists (for exceptions, see Gotthold, 1996; Miller, 1996; Ornstein, 1976). Kohut's ideas have been subject to considerable criticism as well as refinement and modification, and I will not offer a detailed discussion of these controversies. However, Kohut's developmental psychology—his understanding of the child's needs and motivations, and the gradual transformation of these needs in both healthy and pathological development—remains, in my opinion, a profound and essential contribution to our understanding of emotional development in childhood.

In optimal development, the child seeks—and parents provide—affirming responsiveness and sharing of his emergent expressions of interest, joy, pride, and love. Kohut described this fundamental dimension of child development as the child's need for "mirroring" responses to his natural enthusiasms and prideful displays of his developing skills—"the participation of others in these good feelings" (Elson, 1987, p. 71). Mirroring responses are first evident in early exchanges of gaze and smile ("the gleam in the mother's eye") and then vocalizations, between parent and child, and later, in more subdued and selective forms of parental responsiveness. These affirming interactions strengthen the child's feelings of excitement and joy as well as his expansive fantasies and expectations for his future—the child's inner narrative about himself and his sense of what is possible, described by Kohut as aspects of healthy narcissism. In optimal development, parents' increasingly selective responsiveness "transforms crude exhibitionism and grandiosity into adaptively useful self-esteem and self-enjoyment" (Kohut, 1971, p. 284), "a healthy enjoyment of our own activities and successes" (Ornstein, 1978, p. 440). In his classic essay, *Forms and Transformations of Narcissism*, (1966) Kohut proposed that, in healthy development, early forms of narcissism are ultimately transformed into some of our most valuable qualities of character—our capacity for creativity, empathy, humor, wisdom, and the acceptance of death.[5]

In contrast, failure to elicit mirroring responses results in a complex emotional experience Kohut called "fragmentation." Experiences of fragmentation include a broad range of psychological events, from mild embarrassment to severe personality disorganization. These experiences have in common a sense that something is not right, accompanied by feelings of shame (and often rage). When mirroring responses are chronically absent, the child's developing personality will suffer an ongoing vulnerability to narcissistic injuries, and then efforts to hide or compensate for this vulnerability.

Kohut also described a second line of optimal development—a second kind of affirming experiences in childhood that are of critical importance to psychological health. The child derives a feeling of inner strength and well-being from experiences of idealization—being in the presence of, looking up to, and wanting to be like admired adults. The child's idealizations are readily observable to any unbiased observer of young children. In Kohut's theory, these early idealizations are again transformed, through a normally occurring process of gradual disillusionment, into the adult's capacity for commitment to guiding ideals. In pathological development, the child experiences, instead, some form of traumatic disillusionment, leading to cynicism or, in some cases, an urgent search for substitute experiences of idealization.

Experiences of joyful responsiveness and approval from admired adults are sustaining influences in the emotional life of the child. When present, they provide sources of emotional support that facilitate the child's recovery from emotional distress and strengthen what is, again, the critical variable in the emotional health of the child—the child's ability to maintain or restore some good feeling about himself and about others. We observe this healthy development in the child's willingness to seek out and engage in opportunities for joyful interaction, in his readiness to risk the expression of positive affect, and in his quick recovery from frustrations and disappointments.[6]

Lessons from Longitudinal Research

Over the past several decades, longitudinal studies of children at high risk for unfavorable life outcomes have attempted to identify factors that promote successful adaptation despite growing up in conditions of adversity. These studies highlight the decisive importance of the child's *positive expectations for his or her future*—based on the availability of ongoing emotional support. Sroufe et al. (2005), in their presentation of the results of the Minnesota Study of Risk and Adaptation from Birth to Adulthood, argue, for example, that "Resilience is undergirded by unwavering positive expectations regarding self and others (expecting positively even in tough times), flexible self-regulation, and an array of competencies that can be called upon as needed" (p. 227). In this model of development, "a key role is played by [the child's] expectations or representations…expectations and representations are the 'carriers' of experience" (p. 231ff). Sroufe et al. propose that a resilient adaptation to adversity is not based on an inherent quality of the child, but instead, is best understood as an outcome of early, and then ongoing, responsive, supportive care, first evident in the development of a secure attachment relationship. The child establishes patterns of regulation that "become proto-expectations…regarding the external world…with cognitive advances, these expectations are deepened and modified…expectations become beliefs, then attitudes and sophisticated frameworks for interpretation." Sroufe et al. cite Thompson's view that, "In a sense, early experiences (especially with a primary caregiver) help create a 'grammar of emotion' that may be enduring even though the language of emotion continues to unfold in the years to come" (p. 219).

Wyman et al. (1993) also highlight the role of the child's "positive expectations for the future" as a decisive factor in resilient adaptation. In the Rochester Child Resilience Project, "positive future expectations were the most sensitive discriminator" between "stress resistant" and "stress affected" children. Wyman et al. report that positive future expectations "may act as a sustaining counterpoint to the despair that often accompanies chronic stress" and may help a child (like an optimistic adult) persist, rather than give up, in efforts to solve problems; and that "children's positive future expectations related strongly to perceptions of having an involved, nurturant relationship with a primary caregiver" (p. 659). Resilient children developed "expectations of a responsive environment and views of themselves as competent" (p. 659). Wyman et al. cite Werner and Smith's classic description of "a resilient child as one who 'works well, loves well, and *expects* well'" (p. 649).[7]

Paul: "It Stays with Me"

Paul is an intelligent and engaging 10-year-old boy, with a wide range of interests. Paul's parents describe him, from a very early age, as mischievous and impulsive, but also sensitive and sad, given to sullen, dark moods. For long periods of time, Paul seemed generally happy, and in one-on-one interactions with either of his parents, he was enthusiastic, playful, and cooperative. But Paul also "wanted" a lot; he was often relentless in his demands and he could become intensely angry. Although he was a good student, when he became frustrated, Paul would tear up his homework, and he frequently told his parents that he "hates school." Recently, Mr. and Mrs. A. described a "downward spiral" in Paul's mood and behavior. Paul was often angry; he complained that the punishments he received were unfair; and, at times, he expressed the feeling that he was "bad."

I had first met Paul a few years earlier, when Mr. and Mrs. A. consulted me about similar concerns, and I worked with Paul and his parents for a brief period of therapy. Paul played with enthusiasm and he spoke with unusual openness. During these initial meetings, Mr. A. mentioned that Paul often woke up early, and he enjoyed taking a walk with his father to the corner store to buy the morning newspaper. I encouraged Mr. A. to make these early morning walks a daily routine, and both Paul and his father readily agreed. Paul's mood and behavior soon improved—although still mischievous, he seemed more accepting of disappointments and less insistent in his demands.

Mr. and Mrs. A. then called for occasional consultations, when Paul's impulsive or defiant behavior had again caused concern. At these times, Paul was usually happy to talk, at least for a few sessions.

Paul now described recent interactions with his mother. In his own words, he identified a critical pathogenic process: "I don't like the rules... so I'll say something... and she thinks I'm being fresh... and she'll take something away... like my screen time... and that makes me mad... and then *it stays with me*... and she thinks I'm always mad... she says there's a bad vibe in the house... it's a big cycle... when I'm with my friends, it all dissolves away..."

Several months later, I was again talking with Paul. I reminded him of our earlier discussion and how he had described to me the cycle of bad feelings that happens so often in his family—and in many other families. He now added, "You forgot the part where the kid apologizes, but the mom is still angry." With this comment, Paul identified yet another aspect of the pathogenic process—a failure of the child's efforts at repair—and a critical focus of therapeutic intervention.

Julia: "Tell Me There Will Be a Next Time"

Julia's parents had initially consulted me about their 5-year-old daughter. An earlier occupational therapy evaluation had identified significant sensory hypersensitivities, and although Julia was animated, enthusiastic, and talkative once she had warmed up, in new social situations, Julia was shy, often to the point of silence. In a few weeks, Julia would have to take an educational test. Her parents were concerned that, in this unfamiliar setting, Julia would not answer any questions and that no amount of reassurance would alleviate her anxiety. I suggested to Mr. and Mrs. B. that, in the weeks before the test, they create play scenarios with Julia about the upcoming testing encounter.[8] Julia loved this play; each night, she created a different version of the upcoming examination, with different characters ("Mean tester person" or "Nice tester person"), taking turns with her parents in playing different roles. This intervention had been dramatically effective. Julia entered the testing situation with ease and confidence and, in the following weeks, Mr. and Mrs. B. reported a remarkable increase in Julia's willingness to engage in other social encounters—with both adults and peers.

More than a year later, Mr. and Mrs. B. called again. During the past year, the life of this young family had been complicated by serious medical difficulties and economic stress. Now, when Julia came home from school, at the first disappointment of the afternoon, as soon as either of her parents were unable to give her their undivided attention, Julia began to scream—insistent, relentless screaming. Julia's screaming had reduced her intelligent and thoughtful parents to tears. Mr. and Mrs. B. had lost patience with their daughter; their statements and tone with her had become increasingly harsh and punitive. Nothing had helped—ignoring her cries, offering rewards, or imposing "time out" or punishments. Mr. and Mrs. B. sensed that these efforts had only made the situation worse, and they began to doubt their competence as parents. Had they been unable, because of recent family crises, to give Julia enough attention; or, perhaps, in their efforts to compensate for periods of absence and preoccupation, indulged Julia too much?

I suggested to Julia's parents that they enlist Julia in the solution of this problem: to ask her that evening, in a calm moment (perhaps as they were putting her to bed) to tell them about the things that upset her—during the school day and at home. And then, to ask Julia for her ideas—what her parents could say or do to help her when she was upset. This simple "technique" is almost always helpful, even when the solutions children offer are wildly unrealistic or unacceptable. We attempt to engage the child, not in making a protest or a demand, but in finding a solution to an emotional problem. In talking with young children, I sometimes playfully suggest my own implausible solutions: "I think kids should be allowed to stay up as late as they want" or "Let's call the Governor and tell him to pass a law that children should never have to do homework," an implicit challenge to the child to think of a more realistic plan. But I did not anticipate the profound nature of Julia's answer. Julia did not say, "Give me more attention" or "Buy me a toy." Instead, she told her parents, "Tell me there will be a next time."

Julia's parents accepted their daughter's very reasonable suggestion and Julia's emotional crises soon ended. Mr. and Mrs. B. then continued these discussions with Julia. As with Julia's educational test, they began to help Julia anticipate and preview other times when she might begin to feel anxious or angry; they talked together about what Julia could do when her parents were not immediately available to help or comfort her; and they planned special activities that Julia could look forward to, writing them on the calendar. A family atmosphere of escalating anger and defiance gave way to renewed playfulness and emotional support. Julia became increasingly able to tolerate delay and disappointment. And she seemed to "internalize" these discussions; when her mother was upset, Julia would console her, "Mom, it's OK, tomorrow you'll feel better."

***

In my opinion, emotional health and resilience depend, at every stage of life, on the presence of some form of inner or external emotional support that enables us to maintain some good feeling about ourselves and others and some form of positive expectation. I believe this is what Erikson (1959) had in mind when he wrote, in his studies of adolescent identity formation, that a secure sense of identity is accompanied by "the assuredness of anticipated recognition from those who count" (pp. 127–128). As parents, we serve this function for our children throughout life. The child's inner expectation of parental recognition, pride, and approval sustains him during inevitable crises of anxiety, discouragement, and failure. These are critical moments in the emotional life of the child—when admired adults find a way to help a sad, anxious, or angry child realize that this bad feeling will not always be there, that they will not always feel this way. There will be, as Julia said, "a next time." In the absence of this support, the child's experience of painful emotions—and the thoughts, fantasies, and physiological arousal associated with these emotions—remains active and urgent. As Paul explained, "it stays with me."

Notes

1. Panksepp (2001) has presented a similar perspective on emotional health in childhood. "Positive emotional systems appear to operate as attractors that capture cognitive spaces, leading to their broadening, cultivation, and development. Negative emotions tend to constrain cognitive activities to more narrow and obsessive channels" (p. 132). "It cannot be overemphasized that the basic emotional systems may developmentally be like dynamic system attractors that get larger, more complex and more sophisticated as they pull various cognitive structures into their sphere of influence. As a general principle, the larger the sphere of influence of the positive emotions, the more likely is the child to become a productive and happy member of society" (p. 143).
2. Greene, 1998; see also Kramer (2005) on "stuckness" as a characteristic of adult depression.
3. The concept of psychological immunity, I believe, has received insufficient attention in our understanding of both psychopathology and normal development. An exception is Seligman's (1995) cognitive-behavioral program for the prevention of depression in at-risk children, based on the concept of "psychological immunization."

   In a recent report of a dialogue between Western psychologists and Buddhist monks (Goleman, 2003), the Dalai Lama, in his discussion of destructive emotions (what in Buddhism are called "afflictive emotions") refers to the idea of an emotional immune system. The Dalai Lama explained that the development of a well-functioning emotional immune system is a goal of Buddhist meditative practice, enabling the person to resist the afflictive emotions that, like biological pathogens, are an ever-present aspect of our interactions with others. Buddhist meditative practice prescribes a specific "antidote" for each afflictive emotion; in Western child and family psychotherapy, we also have an antidote for the child's destructive emotions—our antidote is empathy.
4. Tronick (2006) explains, "With the experiential accumulation of successful reparations of interactive mismatches, and the attendant transformation of

negative affect and stress into positive affect, the infant establishes a robust positive affective core (Emde, 1983) that biases experience by increasing the likelihood that an event is experienced as positive rather than negative and stressful: in other words, an optimistic, implicit attitude towards events. Importantly, the infant also learns that he or she has control over social interactions" (p. 94).

Schore (1994), in his comprehensive review of the development of affect regulation in infancy, also emphasizes the "internalization . . . of . . . interactive repair transactions" as "critical to the individual's affect regulating capacities for the rest of the lifespan" (p. 241). Demos (1984) has also described, with somewhat older children, reparative sequences of "enjoyment—distress—enjoyment," leading to a general feeling of optimism and confidence.

5. Kohut (1977) argued that the classical psychoanalytic theory of development fails to take into account the joyfulness and pride, normally experienced by both children and parents, that accompanies and supports the child's developmental achievements. More recently, Emde (1991) also observed that, "there is not much Freude (German for joy) in Freud's psychoanalytic psychology" (p. 5). And in clinical writing about children, with some exceptions, healthy development—the importance of positive emotions and the child's need for affirming responsiveness—has received far less attention than pathological processes—the child's negative emotions and his efforts to cope with emotional distress.
6. The seeking of affirming responsiveness in some form continues for all of us throughout life as a basic motivating force and, when present, a sustaining influence. Affirming responsiveness is an important part of what we seek in all our relationships, not only what children seek from parents (and what parents seek from children), but what husbands and wives seek in marriage and what we look for in our friendships. Our need for affirmation may be our most distinctively *human* need. We look for it in the workplace and in all forms of belonging—in the church and in the pub. If we fail to find affirmation in one area of living, we seek it elsewhere, or else we suffer symptoms in the broad sense; or perhaps, in "quiet desperation," we give up and replace the search for affirmation with cynicism or demoralization.
7. In reviewing the findings of the Kauai Longitudinal Study and other studies of successful adaptation in circumstances of high risk, Werner (1995) identified several classes of protective factors that influence positive outcomes. These include: (1) factors within the individual—qualities of temperament that elicit positive responses from caregivers and abilities (for example, scholastic competence or a special interest or hobby the child could share with friends) that provide the child a sense of pride and a belief in his own effectiveness; (2) protective factors within the family—a close bond with at least one competent and emotionally stable person, often a substitute caregiver within the extended family and (3) protective factors within the community—"all of the resilient high-risk children in the Kauai study could point to at least one teacher who was an important source of support" (p. 83).
8. Preoperative therapeutic play has been shown to reduce children's anxiety both prior to and following surgery (Li, Lopez, and Lee, 2007).

3

Theories of Pathological Development: A Brief Review

In Chapter 2, I presented a general theory of optimal and pathological development in childhood. Pathological development was understood to result from negative emotions that *remain active* in the mind of the child and the persistence of modes of thought and behavior associated with negative affects, especially, persistent demands and avoidances. Before I describe, in greater clinical detail, emotional processes that, in interaction with biological risk and vulnerability, eventuate in pathological outcomes in childhood and adolescence, I will offer a brief review of existing models of pathological development in childhood, making note of their strengths and limitations.

Child psychopathology was described by the first generation of child psychoanalysts as a result of psychic conflict, expressed in the form of neurotic symptoms. This early psychoanalytic understanding was then supplemented by a developmental model of pathogenesis—the child's failure to make expected progress along normal developmental lines (for example, from dependence to relative self-reliance, A. Freud, 1974). In a separate tradition, relatively simple behavioral models of child psychopathology were presented that have also been modified and refined (see especially, Granic and Patterson, 2006, discussed below). More recently, cognitive models have been developed, in which the child's moods and problematic behaviors are understood to result from specific cognitive distortions and deficiencies and the construction of maladaptive beliefs. Despite significant theoretical and practical differences in these understandings of development and psychopathology, we should also note some common ground—areas of overlap in a Venn diagram of developmental theories. Contemporary models of pathological development have increasingly focused on the child's capacity for affect regulation as a critical factor in optimal behavioral and emotional adjustment.

Psychoanalytic Theory: The Classical Model

The psychoanalytic understanding of child psychopathology begins with the classical theory presented by Freud, especially in the case of Little

Hans (1909), and reviewed, almost two decades later, in *Inhibitions, Symptoms and Anxiety* (1926). The psychoanalytic theory of psychic conflict provided an understanding of normal and pathological development that remained, until recently, the dominant model of child psychopathology. I will briefly describe this classical theory and offer an appreciation and critique.

In the classical model, the child's symptoms are understood to result from inner conflict and compromise. The result of the child's conflict, whether manifest as symptoms or emerging character traits, is some form of inhibition—an inhibition of the child's curiosity, competitiveness, or self-assertion. These children are often afraid to be openly angry, aggressive, or "bad." They may fear punishment for what they consider to be their bad or unacceptable thoughts (hateful or envious feelings toward parents or siblings, to cite a common example); and, unable to express anger and defiance directly, they express these feelings in disguised form, for example, as frequent somatic complaints or in dreams. In this model, the therapeutic process is understood as the resolution of inner conflict—undoing restrictive defenses and avoidances, lessening irrational anxiety and guilt, and promoting greater freedom of emotional expression. The fundamental aim of these therapeutic measures—an artful blend of interpretation, education, and reassurance—is to expand the child's conscious awareness and acceptance of thoughts and feelings she considers bad or unacceptable, so that normal curiosity and self-assertion can reemerge to replace limiting symptoms and inhibitions. In a review published more than two decades ago, Shapiro and Esman (1985) note that this basic psychodynamic model of child psychopathology and its treatment embodied a "therapeutic core purpose" that "caught the imagination of an entire generation of therapists" (p. 909).

The classical psychoanalytic psychology of childhood remains, in my opinion, an essential contribution to our understanding of normal development, especially the moral development of the child—the child's inner world of being good and being bad, of obedience, and of the child's relation to authority—that forms a core element of every child's character and identity. The unique and outstanding contribution of the classical theory of psychic conflict is the principle of compromise formation: the recognition that all symptoms, in fact, all psychic acts, are overdetermined and must be understood as the product of conflicting motives within the child. A child's behavior, whether normal or symptomatic, will always reflect some expression of conflicting needs and wishes, as the child attempts to reconcile her search for love and affirmation, her aggression and envy, the demands of her conscience, and her need to preserve a feeling of security and self-esteem. In this respect, I believe, the classical psychoanalytic model is correct—only the theory of unconscious conflict, especially the cornerstone concept of defense, allows us to understand the disguised expressions of emotions, needs, and desires that are often part of the child's clinical presentation.[1]

Psychoanalytic Theory: Developmental and Interpersonal Models

Few children, however, present classical "neurotic" symptoms in pure form and the practice of child psychotherapy has required, from the beginning, an alternative model of pathological development and the therapeutic process. Anna Freud (1974) distinguished two types of childhood psychopathology: conflict-based pathology, resulting in symptomatic neuroses and requiring a fundamentally interpretive therapeutic technique, and psychopathology based on "developmental defects," evident in the child's failure to make expected progress along one or more developmental lines, a failure in some aspect of ego development. In Anna Freud's opinion, these children require a different therapeutic approach—now referred to as a program of "developmental help" (Fonagy, 2004)—that includes "admixtures to the [truly analytic] technique such as new positive object attachment, new superego identification, suggestive influence, or even corrective emotional experience which with the very young can set arrested developmental lines going again" (p. 72). Together, the classical and developmental models have provided psychodynamic child therapists with a range of both interpretive and supportive interventions for a wider spectrum of childhood emotional and behavioral disorders.

As a theory of psychopathology, however, especially child psychopathology, conflict theory—even a combined conflict and developmental model—is descriptive, not etiologic (Smith, 2003); that is, these models do not identify factors that initiate and sustain pathological development. Psychoanalytic conflict theory is therefore faced with a fundamental theoretical problem: conflict is universal, but why is *this* child symptomatic? This theoretical dilemma was explicitly recognized by Freud (1926). "Dangers," Freud wrote, "are the common lot of humanity; they are the same for everyone. What we need and cannot lay our finger on is some factor which will explain why some people are able to subject the affect of anxiety... to the normal workings of the mind, or which decides who was doomed to come to grief over that fact" (p. 150). We might ask the same question not only of anxiety but also about sadness, and about envy or shame.[2]

More recently, alternative psychoanalytic theories of child psychopathology models have been proposed. Interpersonal and relational psychoanalytic theories (Altman et al., 2002; Gaines, 1995) have focused on the development of pathogenic relational patterns, restrictive modes of relating, or "false self" adaptations (Winnicott, 1960). In a relational model of child psychotherapy presented by Frankel (1998), for example, psychopathology in childhood is based on the child's need to disavow or dissociate aspects of experience felt as dangerous and the development of rigid, often sadomasochistic, solutions to interpersonal dilemmas. The expressive freedom offered in the therapeutic setting facilitates the enactment, and then eventual integration, of the child's dissociated self-states and a more fully intersubjective mode of interpersonal relationships. Slade (2002) has proposed a model of pathological development, based on attachment theory, in which "aspects of experience, especially affective experience, that preclude the maintenance of attachment relationships are disavowed, reversed, fragmented, or dissociated" (p. 3). Fonagy and colleagues, in a series of important contributions (Bleiberg, Fonagy, and Target, 1997; Fonagy and Target, 1998; Fonagy et al., 2002) have presented an etiological model of severe behavioral and emotional pathology in childhood based on the parents' failure to "mentalize" the child, with consequent impairment of the child's capacity for mentalization and affect regulation.

Self psychology has presented yet another perspective, in which the child's symptoms are understood as experiences of fragmentation or complex sequelae of parental failures of empathy (Gotthold, 1996; Miller, 1996; Ornstein, 1976; Suth, 1996). Pathological development has been described in still other ways: as "the internalization (by the child) of pathological parent-child dynamics" (Oram, 2005) or, in borderline children, as a failure to achieve object constancy and the persistence of primitive defenses, especially splitting, that prevent the maturation and differentiation of object relations (Kernberg, 1983). Mathelin (1999) has presented a Lacanian perspective on child psychotherapy, in which "the child's suffering is a sign that he has a demand but is much too afraid to formulate it" (p. 22) and "things relegated to silence...'murdered'...inside the child...appear in the form of symptoms" (p. 8).

Cognitive and Behavioral Models

Cognitive theories of child psychopathology highlight the therapeutic modification of maladaptive cognitive styles or beliefs (see, for example, Alloy et al., 2001; Reivich et al., 2006; Stark et al., 2008). Kendall (2006) has proposed a frequently cited cognitive framework for understanding child psychopathology: that emotional and behavioral disorders of childhood result from characteristic "cognitive distortions" (for example, a depressed child's belief that she is less capable than other children) and/or "cognitive deficiencies" (for example, an impulsive child's failure to think before acting). Seligman (1995) has presented a cognitive model of childhood depression based on the child's development of pessimistic beliefs. Therapeutic interventions have been developed that attempt to correct cognitive distortions (for example, pessimism or all-or-nothing beliefs) and promote improved emotion-regulation and problem-solving skills. Like psychoanalytic conflict theory, however, most cognitive theories are *descriptive* theories. Cognitive models do not yet account for the origin of pathogenic cognitions: why has the child developed these pathological attitudes, explanations, and beliefs?

Patterson (1982) proposed a highly influential behavioral theory of the pathogenesis of conduct disorders in childhood: that these behavioral disturbances are the outcome of increasingly "coercive" family interactions. Recently, Granic and Patterson (2006) presented an extension and reformulation of coercion theory, based on dynamic systems principles. The revised model includes emotional and cognitive (appraisal) processes in a more complex understanding of coercive interactions. Coercive processes were originally understood on the basis of operant conditioning—parents inadvertently reinforced the child's aggressive or noncompliant behavior by "giving in" to the child's tantrums or refusal. (And parents were reinforced in their capitulation by some momentary respite from the child's demands.) Coercive discipline was also reinforced when a child "gave up" a demand in response to a parent's angry threats ("he only listens when I yell at him"). In the revised theory, Granic and Patterson note that coercive interactions are also characterized by emotion dysregulation, by frequent expressions of anger and contempt, and by increasingly constrained and inflexible patterns of family interactions. They offer an important description of "escalation" processes that typically occur in these families: parents and children develop generalized negative attributions and expectations of each other, and more subtle provocations (for example, a sigh or rolling of the eyes) can initiate angry interactions. Granic and Patterson argue that the revised, dynamic systems model of antisocial development adds subtlety and complexity to our understanding of pathological processes and also provides increased opportunities for therapeutic interventions with children who are at risk for delinquent behavior.

Emotion Regulation: An Emerging Consensus

In recent decades, clinical theory and research, from differing theoretical traditions, has increasingly focused on the importance of affect or emotion dysregulation as a core descriptive feature of child psychopathology (Bradley, 2000; Cole and Zahn-Waxler, 1992; Keenan, 2000). And the child's increasing capacity to regulate the expression of negative emotions has been recognized as a fundamental process in normal development.[3] Both depressed and aggressive children, for example, have been described as lacking effective emotion-regulation skills (Cole and Zahn-Waxler, 1992). In our daily practice, many of the presenting problems of child patients, regardless of diagnosis, can be understood as problems of affect regulation. These children become quickly angry or upset and their expressions of emotional distress are urgent, intense, and prolonged. A child's failure to develop an age-appropriate capacity to "handle" emotions is a common concern of parents and a frequent—perhaps the most frequent—reason for consultation with child clinicians.

Bradley (2000) has proposed that problems of affect regulation are "critical general factors in all major mental disorders" (p. 267). In Bradley's model, which shares important features with the theory presented in this book, constitutional factors (for example, temperament) and environmental factors (for example, insensitive caregiving or trauma) create in the child heightened stress reactivity or prolonged negative affect states. Psychopathology results from maladaptive affect-regulation strategies—strategies focusing on avoidance and affect suppression, leading to internalizing disorders; or oppositional behavior, leading to cycles of negative interactions with caregivers and, later, externalizing disorders. Bradley has also proposed that improved affect regulation is the common factor in all psychotherapeutic treatments, whether cognitive-behavioral, psychodynamic, or pharmacologic.

Cummings and Davies (1995; 1996; Davies and Cummings, 1995) have presented an emotion-regulation model of pathological development in childhood that highlights the role of emotions in organizing children's responses to stressful life events. In the Cumming and Davies model, repeated exposure to stressful events (especially, chronic marital conflict) results in "a general activation of emotion systems and arousal" (p. 126). The child's symptoms reflect the costs incurred by the child in her effort to preserve or restore a sense of emotional security, whether through behavioral withdrawal or active efforts to alter parental behavior.

Cummings and Davies note that, even when they withdraw behaviorally, children do not habituate, or "get used to," marital conflict. Instead, they become sensitized—insecure, hypervigilant, and less able to regulate their emotions. These researchers also report the clinically important finding that while children react to *unresolved* marital conflict with increased emotional and behavioral reactivity—anger, distress, preoccupation, and aggression—marital conflict that is *resolved* elicits little or no distress.

Chorpita (2001) has presented an emotion-regulation theory of anxiety and depressive disorders based on the interaction of biological vulnerability and early experience. In this model, a child's vulnerability to the experience of negative emotions—both anxiety and depression—results from increased (or more easily triggered) activation of a functional brain system that has been labeled the "behavioral inhibition system" (BIS). BIS activity has been proposed as a biological substrate for negative emotions; activation of BIS is characterized by "narrowing of attention, inhibition of gross motor behavior, increased stimulus analysis...increased central nervous system arousal and priming of hypothalamic motor systems for possible rapid action" (p. 113). In the model presented by Chorpita, a child's repeated experience that events are not in her control "amplifies BIS activity in response to events" and results in "a fixed cognitive vulnerability" to experience negative emotions—and therefore increased risk of anxiety or depressive disorders (p. 133).

Several clinical and developmental researchers have proposed that the capacity to regulate emotional impulses effectively depends on the recruitment of "executive" functions. Executive functions are defined as processes that promote the conscious control of thought and action—inhibitory control, planning and problem-solving skills, self-monitoring, a future time orientation, emotion awareness and emotion regulation, attentional capacities, and response flexibility. Greenberg (2006) argues that impaired executive functions are a significant risk factor in the development of antisocial behavior. Greenberg has presented an intervention program for the development of resilience in at-risk youth (PATHS curriculum) based on the development of improved executive functions.

Cognitive-behavioral interventions have also been developed with the goal of promoting emotion regulation and emotional resilience. Reivich et al. (2006; see also Seligman, 1995; Stark et al., 2008) have presented a cognitive-behavioral approach to the development of resilience and a successful treatment program for children and adolescents at risk for anxiety and depression. Reivich et al. note that the thinking of these children is characterized by "a tendency to view one's self, the world, and the future in overly negative ways, combined with a lack of behavioral coping skills" (p. 225). Anxious and depressed children spend more time alone and, when with peers, they engage in more negative interactions. The treatment program developed by Reivich et al. (Penn Resilience Project) attempts to promote emotion regulation and a more resilient adjustment by challenging the child's dysfunctional cognitions (especially a pessimistic explanatory style), teaching problem-solving skills, and facilitating more supportive family relationships. Children are encouraged, for example, to modify negative interpretations and "generate alternative interpretations that are more realistic" (p. 226).

Kovacs et al. (2006) have recently reported a promising pilot study of a cognitive-behavioral treatment program for children with dysthymic disorder (contextual emotion-regulation therapy, or CERT), also based on the development of improved emotion regulation. Kovacs et al. note that, "all empirically supported treatments for depression have components that target aspects of emotion regulation" (p. 900). The authors present an emotion-regulation model of childhood depression. In this model, the child's inability to "down-regulate" (i.e., recover) from distress leads to a "protracted negative mood," which then has adverse affects on both parent-child and peer relationships, leading to "a spiral of symptoms." CERT attempts to teach more effective emotion-regulation responses. Children are taught to identify sources of distress and generate individual emotion-regulation strategies that work for them—active ways of resolving distress, both cognitive (for example, distraction, positive self-talk) and interpersonal (for example, getting a hug). Children and parents watch films together and discuss how characters coped with sadness and distress—what helped the characters feel better and what made them feel worse. They also discuss how to prepare for and cope with negative emotions, to prevent a bad feeling from "getting out of hand."

These interventions to promote resilience illustrate the common ground of contemporary child psychotherapy. A consensus has emerged among clinicians of different schools: that improvement in the child's capacity to regulate emotions is a core component of our therapeutic efforts. And I would note that although the CERT program is labeled a "cognitive-behavioral" intervention, parents and therapists spend considerable time talking with children about the child's bad feelings—what elicits them and what she can do about it.

Notes

1. For excellent clinical presentations of the child's symptoms as compromise formations, see Yanof, 1996, on a case of selective mutism, and Novick and Novick, 1987, on "the essence of masochism."
2. Anna Freud revisited this question a half-century later, with particular reference to children (1974, p. 72): "We have always wondered what determines the *pathogenic impact* (italics in original) of an event. To mention examples: for some children, the birth of a sibling becomes a turning point in development to which all later pathology can be connected; others take this in their stride..." Anna Freud then suggests that the pathogenic impact of a trauma may be determined by the child's progress along relevant developmental lines, for example, toward object constancy or independence in bodily care.
3. In a sense, the contemporary clinical focus on emotion regulation is not new—therapists of all schools, from the beginning, have recognized this essential aspect of emotional health. The psychoanalytic study of affect tolerance begins with Freud's (1911) "Formulations on the Two Principles of Mental Functioning." In this short essay, Freud described what he called a "momentous step" in a child's emotional development: "A new principle of mental functioning was thus introduced; what was presented in the mind was not what was agreeable, but what was real, even if it happened to be disagreeable" (p. 219). In the psychoanalytic literature, affect tolerance and the related capacity for "signal anxiety" are regarded as functions of the ego and indications of ego strength. Important discussions of this aspect of ego development have been presented by Zetzel (1965) on the capacity to "bear" or "master" anxiety and depression, and by Krystal (1976).

4

Psychopathology in Childhood: Malignant and Reparative Processes

A Reparative Perspective

Each of the theories reviewed in the previous chapter highlights an important dimension of pathological development and describes aspects of the complex phenomenology of childhood behavioral and emotional disturbance. Affect dysregulation; inflexible and coercive parent-child interactions; escalation processes; pessimism; impairment of executive functions and lack of social problem-solving skills; all-or-nothing beliefs; restrictive modes of relating; experiences of fragmentation; "silenced" emotions; and emotional conflict are all readily observable in clinical practice with children and families. Often, several of these processes are apparent in a single family.

I would like to propose, however, an alternative perspective on pathological development in childhood—a developmental pathways model that begins with the child's experience of emotional injury and associated painful affects. This perspective highlights processes that are not adequately described by current theories of pathological development, especially, what I believe to be the core pathogenic process in childhood: the development of a demoralized or defiant sense of self. Briefly stated, my thesis is that, in interaction with biological influences, at the core of most child and adolescent psychopathology is an emotional injury that has not been repaired.

For all children, even the most fortunate, some form of emotional injury—experiences of loss or rejection, criticism and disapproval, failure or defeat—are of course, inevitable.[1] And all injuries evoke in the child a complex emotional experience. The child suffers first, a painful affect—comprised, in almost every instance, of feelings of shame, mixed with sadness and anger. At the same time, every injury leads to an intensification of the child's instinctive self-protective responses—some form of withdrawal or retaliatory response (in most cases, some form of both withdrawal and retaliatory response). The child's response to injury is also accompanied, to some degree in every instance I believe, by a restriction in his expression of affect—especially his willingness to risk the expression of positive affect.

In normal, or healthy, development, parents provide for the child some form of reparative emotional experience. Parents (or other adults) who recognize that the child has suffered an injury offer emotional support—solace and encouragement, common understanding, acts of recognition and affirmation, or shared pleasures—that helps the child restore a good feeling about himself and others. Often, a simple acknowledgment of the child's disappointment or frustration is all that is necessary and can accomplish significant repair. In these ways, supportive parents continually repair minor injuries and heal emerging states of demoralization and defiance. And the child's identification with still admired adults—his feeling that he will one day be like those he looks up to—also serves an essential reparative function.

Children, of course, keep many hurts private and hide their painful affects, more or less effectively, even from potentially supportive adults (as perhaps they should, and this contributes to their individuation). Still, these solacing, reparative experiences are important moments in the life of the child. Reparative experiences remain in memory as sources of gratitude and pro-social character development, mitigate the child's "darker" feelings, and become valued elements of identity and character.[2]

Children derive from these repeated experiences of emotional injury, followed by repair, essential aspects of healthy personality development. The child's ability to repair injuries of all kinds—to restore a positive sense of himself and others—is, again, in my view, the critical variable in the emotional health of the child. Successful reparative experiences keep painful affects within a "tolerable" range, allowing ego development and maturing processes to take place, especially, the child's acceptance that disappointments—in himself and others—are part of life, temporary and bearable, leading to some diminution of the urgency of the child's demands. The child learns, in these moments, that being loved survives, that understanding and affirming connections can be restored, and that forgiving and being forgiven are possible, and essential, in all relationships. These maturing processes do not take place in the presence of intense painful affect, when only a narrow focus—on the inner psychic elaboration of painful affects or urgent efforts to get rid of bad feelings—is possible.

Consider, in greater experiential detail, what happens in moments of repair. In these moments, the child feels known and understood. He is therefore less absorbed in defiant thoughts and argument. We have been able, at least in that moment, to arrest the spread of pessimistic attitudes and beliefs (for example, "No one *ever* listens to me," "I am *always* disappointed," "I *always* stink"). We may also have accomplished a reduction in the level of stress hormones and other stress-related physiological processes that have been demonstrated to "poison a child's brain" (Kramer, 2005; Krugman, 2008; Sapolsky, 1996). Behavioral tendencies of withdrawal and defiance are therefore less likely to become established as ingrained pathways, and the child is less likely to develop an angry or demoralized "self," that is, these states of mind do not become core aspects of the child's inner dialogue (Sandler and Sandler, 1998).

The importance of reparative processes has been demonstrated throughout the life span, in Tronick's (1989; 2006) studies of emotional communication in infancy, discussed previously, and in Gottman's (1994) studies of successful marital relationships.[3] Reparative processes, we should note, are present not only at the level of the individual and relationships among individuals, but also at the cellular level—single cells, like the human mind, are involved in continual processes of injury and repair. The efficient functioning of these biological reparative processes is essential to our physical health and survival.[4] In a similar manner, the efficient functioning of *emotional* reparative processes is essential to our *psychological* health and survival. *How well* the child repairs emotional injuries will determine his psychological health or vulnerability to emotional illness. *How* the child responds to injuries, his characteristic modes of repair—that is, the actions of the child's mind and behavior through which he finds solace and affirmation, whether in fantasy, in attitudes, or in active seeking of support from others—will become, in large measure, defining aspects of his character.

When reparative moments are insufficiently present, complex, potentially malignant emotional processes are set in motion. First, a painful affect lingers in the mind of the child. The cognitions (thoughts, attitudes, and expectations), physiological processes, and behavioral tendencies associated with painful affects are strengthened as pathways in the emotional life of the child, and the child enters the next situation—at school, with peers, or at home—ready to be angry, to retaliate, or to withdraw. For these children, or at these moments for all children, the injurious process continues—painful affects and associated fantasies are elaborated in the mind of the child that increasingly color the child's sense of self and others—his attitudes and expectations, his hopes and sense of life's possibilities. In this way, painful emotions become "destructive emotions" (Goleman, 2003).

The child must then search for some way of alleviating these painful affects and restoring some good feeling about himself—some way to feel better. From this perspective, psychopathology in childhood can be understood to result principally from a failure of normal reparative processes. Instead of healing, there is malignancy—a spreading of shame, anger, or sadness in the psyche and failing or maladaptive efforts at self-repair.

Demoralization

These pathogenic processes proceed, in my view, along two basic pathways: (1) a pathway of demoralization, characterized particularly by affects of sadness and shame, evident behaviorally in some form of withdrawal; and (2) a defiant-retaliatory pathway, characterized by anger and grievance. In pathological development, demoralization and defiance become increasingly established as recurrent states of mind, "attractors" in the child's emotional landscape.

In his classic work, *Persuasion and Healing* (Frank and Frank, 1961/1991), Jerome Frank proposed that demoralization was the common characteristic of patients seeking psychotherapy, irrespective of the patient's specific symptoms and diagnosis. Frank also proposed a corollary hypothesis: that the power of the therapeutic relationship to combat or cure demoralization was the common factor in all effective psychotherapies. The concept of demoralization is mentioned infrequently in discussions of child therapy. Still, many of the presenting problems of child and adolescent patients can be understood as expressions of a demoralized self, and Frank's understanding of the syndrome of demoralization in adult patients applies, in many respects, to children as well.

Frank observed that demoralized persons are "conscious of having failed to meet their own expectations or those of others, or of being unable to cope with some pressing problem. They feel powerless to change their situations or themselves." "For many people... [this] distress... is compounded by the feeling that they are somehow unique, that no one else has ever been through a similar experience, and that therefore no one really understands them." "Metaphorically, the demoralized person cowers in a spatiotemporal corner... clings to a small round of individual activities, avoids novelty and challenge, and fears making long term plans." Frank also notes that many patients "successfully conceal their demoralization behind symptoms that seem quite unrelated" (p. 35).

In Frank's understanding, the "major sources of demoralization are the pathogenic meanings patients attribute to feelings and events in their lives" and, in his view, "effective psychotherapies combat demoralization by persuading patients to transform... pathogenic meanings to ones that rekindle hope, enhance mastery, heighten self-esteem, and reintegrate patients with their groups" (p. 52).

All of these features of demoralization apply equally to children—and to the therapeutic process in working with children. In childhood, the "pathogenic meanings" Frank proposed as the source of demoralization are pathogenic feelings and ideas children have developed about themselves and about their effectiveness in the world, what children believe they are able—or unable—to do or to become. And the quality that enables adults to cope with, and even benefit from, stress—what Frank referred to as "stamina"—we now refer to, in childhood, as "resilience."

A child's demoralization may be openly expressed as conscious self-criticism or feelings of low self-esteem; or, when these feelings are denied, reflected instead in his implicit self-attitudes (Conner and Barrett, 2005). In childhood, and especially in adolescence, we recognize demoralization in the form of discouragement, in the child's or adolescent's inability to sustain effort toward goals (or to imagine goals worth working for), in avoidance and giving up, and in diminished affective aliveness, excitement, and joy.

Some degree of demoralization (and some, albeit temporary, experience of shame) follows every academic failure, every competitive defeat, every social rejection, and every failure to elicit expressions of pride and approval from admired adults. As demoralization spreads, the child may come to believe that there is "something wrong" with him, and this shameful feeling is always accompanied, to some extent, by hiding and withdrawal. Demoralization may be evident as pessimism (Seligman, 1995), as a failure of initiative, or as feelings of futility and hopelessness—the child's belief that he cannot change his situation or himself. Many children who are demoralized believe that their parents and teachers make unreasonable demands, leading to feelings of unfairness and resentment. Students with learning disabilities almost universally experience some degree of demoralization. An essential aspect of our therapeutic task is to mitigate or cure the child's demoralization.

Children, of course, do not feel discouraged at every moment, or in every aspect of their lives. Even the most withdrawn child will continue to search to find some good feeling about himself—some place where he can experience a sense of acceptance and of pride. Because they are less able to sustain effort, however, demoralized children are likely to seek pride and acceptance in activities that provide an *immediate* good feeling—a good feeling that does not have to be worked for. For some children, this may be, in part, the appeal of video games, and, in adolescence, the appeal of risk-taking and antisocial behavior, and of substance abuse.

Defiance

A child's expressions of defiance may also take many forms. Defiance begins as some form of *protest* or refusal. In pathological development, the child's instinctive defiant response to painful affects—saying "No" in response to an experienced or anticipated frustration—is strengthened, leading to increasingly unyielding attitudes and behavior. Like demoralization, a child's defiance may be expressed openly (for example, in oppositional behavior, in not speaking, or in lying) or covertly, in the child's attitudes and imagination (for example, as cynicism or as fantasies of revenge). Defiance is often expressed as stubbornness or argument and as sarcasm and "disrespect." Defensiveness (a form of argument and an instinctive response to criticism) is a very common expression of defiance. Parents who argue frequently with their children engender increased defensiveness in the child. Typically, these arguments produce no increase in compliance with parental requests; instead, children simply become good at arguing.[5]

A child who is publicly ridiculed by his teacher (or privately ridiculed by a parent) may not say "Fuck you" to his parent or teacher; but he will think "Fuck you," and this attitude—if it remains active—will find some expression in his imagination or behavior, perhaps as disparagement or contempt, or, at some later time, displaced against more vulnerable others, in bullying; or against groups of others, in bigotry. (This common process has been understood in classical psychoanalytic psychology as "identification with the aggressor.") Persistent defiant attitudes result, ominously, in an inner destruction of parental influence and authority ("I don't care what he thinks"). Although the waning of parental authority is a normal phase of development in mid-to-late adolescence, this process is pathological when it occurs in childhood.[6]

An impulsive temperament is a significant risk factor for the development of defiant modes of thought and behavior. Impulsive children become more quickly angry and also have greater difficulty inhibiting instinctive defiant responses. This quality of temperament therefore places increased demands on the emotional maturity of parents and teachers, who are more likely to react harshly to the child's defiant behavior, setting in motion the common defiant cycle of interaction.

As clinicians, when we evaluate the severity of a child's or adolescent's psychological disturbance, we make some judgment about how extensive—and how unyielding—the child's demoralization and defiant attitudes have become. How quickly does this child bounce back from disappointments? How extensively have resentment and grievance spread? Is he able, under some circumstances, to show enthusiasm and initiative; to express positive, realistic expectations; and to acknowledge the needs of others? This intuitive assessment will then influence our recommendations to parents, especially about the intensity and length of treatment that will be required.

In my clinical experience, some degree of *both* demoralization and defiance are ordinarily present in the emotional lives of troubled children, implicit in many common complaints ("I hate school"; "I hate my teachers"; "I hate my life"). And what Frank proposed with respect to adult patients is, I believe, also true of children: that a core feeling of demoralization, often silent or actively denied, and expressed in myriad forms, is at the heart of what most troubles most children.

Vicious Cycles

Pathological development in childhood typically proceeds in escalating, vicious cycles of negative interactions. A child's impulsive, immature, or "difficult" behavior elicits angry and critical reactions from parents and teachers, and often from peers. (The child may overhear other children saying, "Don't play with Jeremy, he's annoying.") These critical responses reinforce the child's sense of injury. He feels badly about himself and angry at others, and he is now more likely to withdraw from peer interactions, to persist in his immature behavior, or to respond, either in the present or at some later time, with increased defiance. He may begin to act "weird" or provocative with peers, or to think of himself as one of the "bad" kids; and he may retaliate, in fantasy or with overt actions that perpetuate a vicious cycle of anger and alienation.

Parental criticism and peer rejection evoke in the child a bad feeling about himself that is difficult to get rid of. When we are able to glimpse the inner world of these children, perhaps through their writings, drawings, or fantasy play, we find that many of them have developed an emotional life dominated by feelings of shame and envy, and fantasies of revenge against those who have hurt or rejected them.

The Role of Conflict

Because of the historical—and continuing—importance of the theory of psychological conflict in understanding child psychopathology, I would like to return to the question posed by Freud and Anna Freud—if childhood conflicts are universal, why is this child symptomatic?—and offer a perspective on the role of conflict in normal and pathological child development. Conflict (whether the instinctual and moral conflicts of Freud's theory or conflicts among "relational configurations" in Mitchell's [1988] relational-conflict theory) is always present in the emotional life of the child. In this respect, Freud's theory is correct—when we are able to be sufficiently introspective and honest with ourselves, we will find conflict to be continuously present and a determining force in our lives. How a child resolves the universal conflicts of childhood is decisive in shaping the child's character—what kind of person he will become. Some character adaptations are overly restrictive: a child, for example, may become excessively obedient or "good," or overly dependent, or cover over a core feeling of shame with a bravado of superiority. These character traits may not work well for the child at later stages of his life, limiting his choices or undermining the quality of his love and work relationships. In childhood, the feelings and fantasies associated with emotional injuries *intensify* the child's conflicts—retaliatory and envious fantasies, for example, may evoke or intensify conscious or unconscious feelings of guilt or fear of punishment.

A child's character will then determine the ultimate expression of his symptoms, that is, in what form his demoralization, protest, or grievance is expressed—*how* a child expresses sadness or anger, whether overt or disguised (even from himself). And the therapist's understanding of the child's conflicts is a necessary aspect of therapeutic work with many children. Still, in the model of pathological development I have proposed, in childhood and most often in adolescence as well, conflict is not the primary pathogenic agent. These children are too sad or too angry in the first place.[7]

With this model of optimal and pathological emotional development as a guide, I will now consider the process of therapeutic change: how can we best promote in children a more resilient adjustment, a more confident and joyful participation in life.

Notes

1. In contemporary practice, it is important to keep in mind that not all emotional injuries originate in family relationships. For many children, especially the child with a learning disability, daily life in the classroom, and often on the playground, inflicts severe injuries to the child's self-esteem, in the form of peer rejection and academic failure. Some degree of academic difficulty—the result of even mild-moderate attention or learning disorders, with consequent discouragement and frustration—may be the most common risk factor for all forms of child psychopathology. In an epidemiological survey of childhood emotional and behavioral problems (Achenbach et al., 1991), difficulty with schoolwork was the most commonly reported symptom. A combination of academic failure and parental scorn places the child at enormous risk for depression and/or anti-social development and may be a lethal mixture for many adolescents.
2. Older children, and adolescents especially, will seek sources of solace outside the family. In childhood, and throughout life, the sense of well-being that comes from belonging to a supportive community, from participation in traditions of all kinds, or from spiritual practice, also serves a reparative function. The decline of these societal sources of emotional support is frequently cited as a possible causal factor in the increased prevalence (epidemic) of depression and related disorders reported over the course of recent decades (see, for example, Seligman, 1995).
3. Gottman reports that normal repair mechanisms—repair processes that usually occur during marital conflict (for example, humor or finding areas of common ground)—"do not work in ailing marriages" (1994, p. 416). The couple is therefore more likely to enter an "absorbing state" of "negative affect reciprocity" and less able to interrupt a "cascade" of negative interactions—criticism, contempt, defensiveness, and stonewalling—that predicts divorce.
4. The mechanisms of cellular damage and repair and the pathogenic effects of inactive reparative mechanisms are widely studied biological processes. "DNA repair is regarded as one of the essential events in all life forms" (Dizdar et al., 2003). For theoretical reviews, see Maier and Watkins (1998) and Matzinger (2002).
5. Popular programs that help parents argue less with their children—and listen more (for example, Ginott, 1965; Nichols, 2004)—and then assert parental authority with greater clarity (for example, Phelan, 1995) are therefore of great value to many families.
6. In the psychoanalytic tradition, Harry Stack Sullivan (1953) proposed that children develop a hostile and suspicious attitude towards others—the belief "that one really lives among enemies"—when the child, at moments when he is in need of tenderness, is "treated in a fashion to provoke anxiety or even, in some cases, pain" (p. 214). Sullivan referred to this process as a "malevolent transformation." Winnicott (1956) described similar defiant processes—what he called "hate products in the psyche"—in his analysis of the antisocial tendency.

7. This perspective also suggests an answer to Anna Freud's question regarding the pathogenic impact of injurious or traumatic events in the life of the child: that the impact of traumatic events will depend, most critically, on the capacity of the child *and his or her supportive environment* to effect some repair—to prevent the spread of painful affects and fantasies and enable the child to recover a positive sense of self. (For a related, but somewhat different, answer to Anna Freud's question, see Tyson and Tyson, 1990.)

Part II

The Therapeutic Process

5

The Therapeutic Process: An Overview

Review: The Basic Model

In the preceding chapters, I have presented an emotion-based perspective on optimal and pathological development in childhood. From this perspective, psychological health is characterized by a predominance of positive emotions and positive expectations—an expansion of thoughts and fantasies (or scripts, or beliefs) associated with the affects of interest, excitement, joy, pride, and love. In emotional health, the child develops the capacity to bounce back from emotional injuries and restore a positive feeling about herself and her future. We call this *emotional resilience*, or psychological immunity.

In contrast, pathological development is characterized by an elaboration or strengthening, in the mind and behavior of the child, of beliefs and action tendencies associated with painful affects—feelings of anger, shame, anxiety, and sadness. Painful emotions *remain active* in the mind of the child; the child's emotional life is characterized by qualities of *urgency* and *inflexibility* and her interactions with parents, teachers, and peers increasingly take the form of vicious cycles—of criticism and defiance; anger, exclusion, and withdrawal. In pathological development, negative emotions have become habitual and pervasive, deep "attractors" in the child's emotional landscape.

In the following chapters, I will present a perspective on therapeutic work with children and families based on these principles of emotional health and illness. In the therapeutic setting, we attempt to set in motion a process of repair. The guiding principle of our work will be to strengthen processes, in children and in families, that foster resilience—to arrest the spread of malignant events in the mind of the child, strengthen the child's expectation of affirming responsiveness, and restore more optimistic beliefs about her future.

Engagement

The first task of any effective clinical work with children is to engage the child in a process of open communication—therapeutic play or talk. Children, however, are famously resistant, and often respond to the most tactful inquiries—from their most warm and accepting therapists—by telling us, "I don't remember" or "I don't know." In my experience, we most successfully engage children in some form of therapeutic dialogue or interaction by adopting two fundamental attitudes: (1) our empathic recognition of the child's distress and *grievance* and (2) equally important, the therapist's enthusiastic, affirming responsiveness to the child's interests and positive affects. These processes of engagement are more than a preparatory phase of building rapport; they are also beginning processes of therapeutic change. When we are able to engage a child in animated, responsive play and listen patiently to a child's grievance—and, better yet, when we are able to help parents engage more frequently with their children in these ways—we often observe rapid improvement in a child's mood and behavior.

Understanding

Engagement, however, is not yet understanding, and for most children and families, there are still significant obstacles to therapeutic success. Having engaged the child in animated interaction, the child therapist is now faced with a fundamental question about the process of therapeutic change: What kind of understanding is helpful to children? In psychodynamic approaches to child therapy, the development of insight or self-understanding, conveyed in the therapist's interpretations of the child's play, dreams, or interactions with her therapist, has traditionally been considered a central mechanism of therapeutic change. But the question of how a child makes use of insight is problematic. Interpretative "moments" (Pine, 1985) are both difficult to achieve and then of uncertain therapeutic effect. Experienced psychodynamic child therapists regularly report that their interpretations to children are often simply ignored—or worse, misconstrued as criticisms, leading to severe, iatrogenic resistances. If the path from insight to change is often obscure in work with adult patients, it is much more so with children. The failure of understanding, by itself, to produce observable change in children has been a source of dissatisfaction to both parents and child therapists and an impetus for the development of more active, performance—based, behavioral and cognitive-behavioral approaches to the treatment of children.[1]

It may be helpful to recall the goal of interpretation and insight in the classical model of psychoanalytic child therapy. In the classical model, therapeutic change results from an expansion of the child's emotional life by bringing into the child's awareness—and helping the child tolerate—threatening affects and ideas. Sugarman (1994), for example, suggests that interpretation of the child's conflicts "promotes increased acceptance of previously disavowed mental contents" and, in this way, "facilitates a developmentally more advanced self-representation" (or, in Roy Schafer's [1999] felicitous phrase "an enriched version of self").[2]

In practice, psychoanalytic child therapists developed a broadened understanding of the therapist's interpretive function—from the goal of promoting conscious knowledge and acceptance of unacceptable wishes (making the unconscious conscious) to helping children become familiar with a greater range of feelings. In this model, the therapist's interventions focus on the recognition and naming of affect states (Katan, 1961), whether expressed in the child's play or discussion of life events—the therapist's recognition, for example, of the child's unacknowledged feelings of sadness, worry, or anger, or wish to be cared for. In the psychodynamic tradition, this is the child therapist's most basic and most obvious therapeutic function—helping children talk about bad feelings.

This therapeutic model still applies to many children, perhaps to most children at some time in the course of therapy—when we are able to help a child express emotions she has held back, and then show her how these feelings have been expressed in some other form, how her holding back of feelings has lead to symptoms and inhibitions. It soon became apparent, however, that this basic therapeutic process, although important, was not a *sufficient* model of therapeutic change—other therapeutic processes were necessary.

The practice of psychodynamic child psychotherapy has therefore required an alternative therapeutic model, based not on the therapist's *interpretive* function, but instead on the therapist's role as a "new object" or "auxiliary ego," fostering aspects of ego development, for example, reality testing and impulse control, and more recently, "mentalization" (Fonagy and Target, 1998; Fonagy et al., 2002). This model of child therapy, increasingly influenced by attachment theory and research, was developed especially at the Anna Freud Centre in London and is referred to as a therapy of "developmental help" (Fonagy, 2004). Consistent with this understanding of therapeutic change, Sugarman (2003) has proposed that child therapy promotes not "insight," but rather, "insightfulness," that is, increased capacity to "mentalize" experience, with consequent improvement in the child's capacity for affect regulation.

Psychodynamic (and humanistic) child therapists have also recognized the therapeutic potential of play with an empathic, responsive therapist, often accompanied by minimal interpretation and insight, in promoting the child's sense of mastery, inner coherence, and capacity for symbolization (see, especially, Slade, 1994; also Cohen and Solnit, 1993; Drucker, 1994; Frankel, 1998). In this therapeutic model, "simply playing" (Slade, 1994) serves a noninterpretive, developmental function, helping the child create an increasingly complex inner world and more modulated expression of affect. All therapists who play with children have experienced this important, but still poorly understood, therapeutic result: that a child's mood and behavioral adjustment may improve dramatically, based on something *experiential,* something that *happens,* in the course of therapeutic play that is not necessarily verbalized.

From the beginning, therefore, the importance of relationship factors and supportive interventions in work with children have been generally acknowledged as essential to therapeutic success and to "peacefully coexist" (Pine, 1985; see also Chethik, 2000; Shapiro and Esman, 1985) with the task of interpretation.

Emotional Understanding: The Role of Empathy

With this brief introduction in mind, I would like to propose a framework for the role of understanding in child psychotherapy. In my opinion, the first and most fundamental understanding we offer children—and our most potent therapeutic intervention or "technique" to promote resilience and psychological immunity—is *empathy*. Although empathy is universally acknowledged as an essential component of all successful psychotherapy, the role of empathic understanding in child therapy remains, I believe, insufficiently appreciated, perhaps taken for granted.

The language of therapeutic communication with children is first and foremost a simple empathic language of affect and intention—of having "good feelings" and "bad feelings," of wanting and not wanting, of feeling sad or angry, frustrated and disappointed. In my personal clinical experience, of all the things we say to children and parents in the course of treatment, it is our simple empathic communications that have the most palpable effect. And these empathic statements are often noteworthy, as Fonagy and Target (1998) have written, for their qualities of "ordinariness and humanity."

I will present a specific hypothesis on the therapeutic function of empathy in clinical work with children: that empathic understanding *arrests the spread of painful emotions* in the mind of the child and reduces the urgency and inflexibility that are characteristic of pathological emotional states. In moments of empathic understanding, as we all know from personal experience, anger subsides, and sadness and shame are attenuated. Empathic understanding promotes reduced stress at the physiological level and increased flexibility at the cognitive—emotional level. Behaviorally, we see less withdrawal, less defiance, and less argument.

Experiences of empathic understanding ("being heard") then allow maturing processes to take place—the child becomes, in small increments, more open to educative and socializing influences, to compromise, and active problem-solving. In this way, empathic understanding promotes a decisive change in the child's attitudes and behavior and facilitates a fulcrum shift in emotional development—away from urgent and insistent demands and toward tolerance for disappointments and frustrations, and acceptance of personal responsibility.

Understanding and Action: The Child's Defenses

These are profoundly therapeutic processes. But empathy is not enough. As part of their repertoire of instinctive self-protective mechanisms, children often hide their painful affects, from others and from themselves, giving rise to stubborn resistance to those who seek to help. Most children, when referred for treatment, have already constructed rigid systems of demands and avoidances, buttressed by inner argument. Our task becomes especially complex when malignant processes have developed extensively, influencing core aspects of the child's inner world and external adaptation. And it is an undeniable clinical fact that children often do not want to talk about their bad feelings (and, especially, their bad behavior).

Successful treatment of children therefore requires, in most cases, a second phase of therapy: we need to challenge children—still guided by our understanding of the child's emotions—to think or act differently, perhaps in ways they had not thought of, or have refused to do. Many children referred for psychotherapy, even children who are primarily withdrawn, require some improved socialization—improved behavioral control or improved peer relationships. These children need to learn to control their aggression, to play by the rules, and to be able to make and keep friends.

In this phase of therapy (or at these moments) we offer a different kind of understanding—and explicit encouragement for behavioral change. We talk with children not only about how they feel or about what evoked their bad feelings, but also about what they *do* with their bad feelings—what children *do*, and can do differently, when they feel angry, disappointed, or worried. In this way, we provide a form of insight—about the links between affect and behavior—and increased awareness of the child's self-protective strategies, her efforts to get rid of bad feelings.

And we present some incremental challenge to the child's avoidant or defiant modes of coping with negative emotions. We encourage children to develop less restrictive modes of thinking and relating—a new sense of what is possible. The function of this phase of the therapeutic process is to unlock some form of rigidity, for example, stubbornness—whether stubborn avoidance or stubborn defiance. We promote, in this way, more mature means of coping with (i.e., regulating) painful affects—the child is now able to *be* angry, anxious, or sad without withdrawal, defiance, or explosive action.

At this point in the treatment process, behavioral and cognitive-behavioral interventions are helpful and often necessary. Effective therapeutic work with children often requires active efforts on the part of the therapist to modify dysfunctional cognitions (Kendall, 2006), especially pessimistic evaluations of self (Seligman, 1995); to teach active problem-solving (e.g., Kendall, Aschenbrand, and Hudson, 2003; Kovacs et al., 2006; Stark et al., 2008); and to promote, through positive reinforcement, more adaptive, pro-social behavioral responses (Kazdin, 2005). Successful programs for the treatment of children with anxiety, depression, or aggressive behavior encourage children to think and act differently when faced with painful feelings. These interventions challenge children to develop greater acceptance of frustrations and disappointments and more mature expressions of anger and distress; to play without cheating; or, for anxious children, to try new things and "expand their comfort zones." And we offer encouragement and praise for each advance in the child's progress toward these goals.

Parent Guidance

There is no inherent reason that parents cannot be partners in these therapeutic processes. In contemporary practice, some form of parent counseling—especially to promote enhanced parental sensitivity and parental competence (Bleiberg, Fonagy, and Target, 1997)—is considered essential to successful treatment by child therapists of all schools. The regular inclusion of parents in the treatment process, whenever possible, is perhaps the most pervasive change in the practice of child therapy, and our inability to maintain a working alliance with parents is commonly acknowledged as a frequent cause of therapeutic failure. Child therapists have always offered both common sense and theoretically-informed guidance to parents; with recent advances in our understanding of children's emotional development, we may now be able to do much more.

Families of troubled children are "stuck"—locked in frequent angry, and increasingly despairing, patterns of interaction. Both parents and children have come to feel justified in their anger and resentment. Parents are often dismissive of their child's feelings and (at times, with some justification) regard the child's behavior and expressions of emotion as in some way ungenuine—"manipulative" or "controlling." Children, for their part, have become secretive, defensive, and often untruthful, and harbor feelings, especially, of unfairness.

The repair of parent-child relationships is therefore a goal of almost every consultation and treatment. Beginning in the initial consultation, we attempt to identify and ameliorate pathogenic patterns of family interactions—vicious cycles that perpetuate defiance and withdrawal—and strengthen affirming responsiveness between parents and their children. In the course of this work, when we are able to effect some repair of family relationships that have been damaged by frequent anger and resentment; when we are able to help parents cope with the demands of being a parent and take greater pleasure in their children; and when we are able, regardless of the child's presenting symptoms, to help restore some measure of joyfulness that has been lost or eroded in the lives of the parents and children who consult us, we should certainly count this as a measure of therapeutic success. In the end, these salutary changes in parent-child relationships may be the most important—and lasting—benefits of our therapeutic efforts.

Diagnosis and Assessment: Essential Diagnostic Questions

We begin with a diagnostic evaluation. The value of our current diagnostic categories (and, more generally, of categorical versus dimensional approaches to the diagnosis of childhood emotional and behavioral problems) remains controversial, and a discussion of these complex issues is beyond the scope of this book. Clearly, most of the problems presented to us by parents—whether problems of attention, mood, or behavior—exist on a continuum of severity, and diagnostic discriminations are therefore often arbitrary. It is generally recognized, for example, that a child who does not meet diagnostic criteria for an attention or learning disorder is not very different from a child who does meet current diagnostic criteria.

In other cases, however, discrete diagnosis is essential. Diagnosis is essential when (1) adjunctive therapies are necessary as part of a comprehensive treatment program and (2) identification of a specific disorder contributes to our understanding of the complex etiological factors and developmental pathways that lead to a child's emotional or behavioral disturbance.

These are the critical diagnostic questions that child therapists must consider before beginning any therapeutic intervention—and our most common diagnostic errors:

(1) Does This Child Have a Learning Disability?

The failure of schools and mental health professionals to identify and provide adequate remedial intervention to children with learning disorders, although now less frequent than a generation ago, remains a relatively common—and egregious—error. My clinical experience over several decades, in hospital, residential, and out-patient settings, justifies the following recommendation: *Every* child whose parents or teachers report ongoing resistance to completing schoolwork or homework; *every* child whose performance in school is below expectations based on his parents' or teachers' intuitive assessment of his intellectual potential; and *every* child who, over an extended period of time, complains that he "hates school" or "hates reading" should be evaluated for the presence of an attention or learning disorder *even when other possible pathogenic processes (for example, marital conflict, divorce, or medical illness) are also present.* We need to be especially alert to the presence of subtle, "low severity—high prevalence" difficulties in learning (Levine, 1987) that are a significant source of anxiety, frustration, and demoralization for children—and conflict in parent-child relationships.

These children are not "lazy." (Mel Levine's book, *The Myth of Laziness, 2003*, should be required reading for all clinicians working with children and families.) A "diagnosis" of "laziness," however, is still unfortunately common. I frequently explain to parents that, as psychologists, "lazy" (and, especially, "just lazy") is not in our dictionary. At best, lazy is a description in need of an explanation. In most cases, we will replace this description with a different understanding: that the child is anxious, discouraged, frustrated, or angry.

A diagnosis of laziness leads to only one prescription: the child must "try harder"; and this incorrect understanding then leads, almost inexorably, to family conflict and increasing demoralization and defiant moods. For children with learning difficulties of all kinds, doing their homework is like running with a sprained ankle—it is possible, although painful. And the child, like all us, will find ways to avoid or postpone this painful (and discouraging) task. Or she may run ten steps and then find a reason to stop. Parents and teachers may tell us that the child "can do it when she tries" and there is some truth in this observation. We cannot run, of course, if we have a broken ankle; but most learning disabilities are more like sprains than fractures. On some occasions, therefore, when the intrinsic interest, or anticipated success, or encouragement, or promise of material reward is great enough, the child will overcome her frustration and put forth effort in the task—but she cannot do this every time or every day.

In my experience, the identification of learning disorders has often been delayed for several years because schools and clinicians have made the *assumption* that the child's resistance to schoolwork was based on emotional factors. During this time, families have pursued unsuccessful psychotherapeutic interventions, parent-child conflict over schoolwork has remained unabated, and children have failed to receive appropriate remedial intervention, increasing their demoralization and anger.

It is therefore essential to accurately diagnose learning disorders—to identify the child's areas of academic difficulty and provide remedial intervention. It is equally important, however, to appreciate and nurture the child's strengths. In school, children are expected to perform well in all academic subjects. In life, it is more important for us to excel in one area of endeavor. I am frequently consulted by parents whose children, now adolescents, have been accurately diagnosed with some form of learning disability and provided with appropriate academic remediation and accomodations. Unwittingly, however, parental attention toward improving the child's academic deficits has had a serious side effect: highlighting the child's awareness of her weaknesses, rather than her strengths, and promoting in the child a feeling that there is "something wrong" with her; and she has become increasingly discouraged and angry.[3]

Children with learning disabilities *always* experience frequent moments of frustration and discouragement. Many suffer chronic feelings of shame and low self-esteem, at times masked by defensive or defiant attitudes. As adolescents, many of these children continue to feel that they are "not smart," despite considerable talents, areas of academic competence, and interpersonal skills that will serve them well in life. Recently, in talking with children and adolescents I have evaluated for possible learning disorders, or children I am working with in psychotherapy, I have made literal use of our theoretical concept of "self-image" or "self-representation." I tell the child (and explain to parents) that I am going to draw a picture of her. I then draw a blank rectangle and explain what should be in the center of the picture: the child's strengths—her friendships; her athletic or musical or artistic or dramatic talents; her understanding, reasoning, and problem-solving abilities—and I draw in the corner, not the center—her weaknesses, perhaps a difficulty with math or writing, or that, right now, she needs some help in reading. This exercise seems simplistic, even a little contrived; often, however, this is not how children—or their parents—have come to see themselves. We need to help these children change their picture of themselves to one in which their strengths are in the center and their weaknesses are in the corner, not, as is so often the case, the other way around.

(2) Does This Child Have ADHD or Qualities of Temperament on the ADHD Spectrum?

Whether medicine or nonmedical treatment methods are used at any point in the child's life, the identification of an attention deficit-hyperactivity disorder (ADHD) often profoundly changes a family's understanding of their child. This new understanding—again, that the child is not lazy or malicious but, instead, has more difficulty than other children initiating or sustaining focused attention on certain tasks or inhibiting undesired behaviors—helps many parents respond with greater empathy and patience to a child's problematic behaviors and, in this way, alters the course of pathological development.

(3) What Other Qualities of Temperament—for example, Behavioral Inhibition, Negative Emotionality, Problems of Sensory Integration or Motor Coordination—Have Contributed to the Child's Withdrawn or Defiant Behavioral Tendencies and to the Development of Destructive Patterns of Parent-Child Interactions?

The contribution of a child's temperament to family relationships and the role of temperament as a risk or protective factor in the development of child psychopathology is one of the most widely recognized facts of clinical child psychology (Wachs, 2006)—and a first lesson learned by beginning child therapists in listening to parents describe their children. A parent's appreciation of a child's temperament is often of critical importance. This understanding not only relieves inappropriate parental guilt, but also permits a more empathic understanding of the child—and therefore a more constructive response to the child's problematic moods and behaviors.

(4) Does this Child Have a Biologically-based Anxiety or Mood Disorder, Especially OCD?

The prominence of biological factors in the development of most severe anxiety disorders in childhood, especially obsessive-compulsive disorder (OCD), is also now well established (March, Leonard, and Swedo, 1995). Child therapists must be familiar with both the typical as well as less common symptoms of OCD in childhood. Failure to recognize the varying manifestations of OCD or PANDAS (Swedo et al., 1998) in children remains a relatively frequent diagnostic error. Cognitive-behavioral therapy—often in combination with medicine—*not* psychodynamic or emotion-based psychotherapy—is the treatment of choice for OCD in childhood. Of course, children with OCD may also present other emotional or behavioral difficulties, or problems in family or peer relationships. They may be demoralized and angry for reasons unrelated—or related in complex ways—to their OCD; these children will then benefit from the emotional support described in subsequent chapters. It is essential, however, to recognize OCD as a discrete disorder, requiring specialized treatment.

The identification of mood disorders in childhood is our most difficult diagnostic challenge. Unlike ADHD and OCD, childhood bipolar disorder has few readily identifiable pathognomonic symptoms; it is therefore very difficult to distinguish bipolar disorder from problems of mood regulation caused by a combination of other factors, or even from mood lability experienced at some time by many children. On this diagnostic issue, I will offer only my personal clinical experience and a note of caution. The identification of bipolar disorder in children is a significant advance in psychiatric diagnosis. Problems of emotion regulation, however, are very common among children. These problems result from the interaction of multiple causes and can most often be successfully treated with individual and family therapy. Childhood bipolar disorder, requiring psychopharmacological treatment, although present in some cases, is uncommon; and the dramatic increase in clinicians making this diagnosis and prescribing medicines for these children—before any psychotherapeutic interventions have been attempted—is alarming.

* * *

Our assessment of every child includes these essential diagnostic questions, but then goes beyond diagnosis. For each child, we attempt to develop working hypotheses of the origins and sustaining factors that contribute to the child's emotional distress and behavioral disturbance—to identify the multiple pathogenic factors that interact to determine the child's presenting problems.

As conflict models of psychopathology have given way, at least in part, to developmental pathways models, we now have a greater appreciation of the role of both biology and family processes in children's emotional and behavioral problems. Regularly, we find a biological factor or factors, especially behavioral inhibition (Biederman et al., 1993) or disinhibition (Barkley, 1997a), some form of difficult temperament or learning disorder. In most cases, we also find some contributing, or exacerbating, family or social factors, especially, inflexible patterns of parent-child interactions or peer rejection.

It is especially important to identify patterns of family interactions that sustain a pathogenic process. We inquire, therefore, not only about the history of the family, but also about current family relationships. Even when there have been traumatic events in the life of a family, we need to alter current, "real-time" (Granic and Patterson, 2006) parent-child interactions. This inquiry is not always easy. The child's (and parents') defensiveness not only makes change difficult, but often obscures the nature of their interactions. Finally, we include in our assessment an appreciation of the child's individual strengths—her talents and qualities of character and personality—as well as her vulnerabilities.

Having made these assessments, we will be in a better position to present to parents an initial recommendation about how we can help—at what points in a complex pathway of ongoing, potentially pathogenic, events we can most effectively intervene. My own work includes, in almost every case, both individual child therapy and parent guidance. The structure and frequency of therapy—how often a child is seen individually, or jointly with a parent or parents, and how often parents are seen alone—varies with the needs of each child and family. These decisions are not based on a priori rules, but, instead, on how we can best achieve our initial therapeutic goals. In what setting are we most likely to mitigate the child's anxiety and resistance and establish a therapeutic dialogue? And how urgent is the need to begin to repair destructive family relationships? We then initiate a therapeutic process: an effort to arrest the spread of malignant emotions, strengthen the child's initiative and problem-solving, and promote more affirming parent-child interactions.

Notes

1. We can, of course, go farther and ask, "Is understanding necessary at all?" In some traditions of child therapy, insight—the child's increased understanding of herself—plays a small role in the process of therapeutic change. Behaviorist models explicitly eschew self-understanding as a mechanism of change. Insight also plays a limited role in the humanistic tradition of child therapy (Axline, 1947; Moustakis, 1997; Wright, Everett, and Roisman, 1986). Humanistic child therapy offers, instead, a model of the therapeutic process based on the establishment of a special therapeutic relationship; the therapist's primary task is not to provide understanding, but—through acceptance and empathy—to reach, and create engagement with, a withdrawn or angry child. Cognitive approaches to child therapy offer the child a specific kind of understanding—how thinking influences feeling—in an effort to modify the cognitive biases and distortions that evoke and sustain maladaptive emotional responses.
2. Sugarman cites Arlow's opinion that, through insight, a patient in psychoanalysis "comes to understand how his mind works" (1994, p. 330). In a related formulation, Chethik (2000) defines the therapist's interpretative function as "to give meaning to behavior that is controlled by unconscious processes" (pp. 120–121).
3. Brooks (2006), based on a similar understanding, recommends that parents actively nurture the child's "islands of competence."

6

Therapeutic Engagement

All effective clinical work with children begins with the engagement of the child in a process of open communication—therapeutic play or talk. The child therapist's first task is therefore to cultivate a way of being with children—and with each individual child—that facilitates the child's expression of emotion, in his own individual style. With some children, engagement is a relatively simple matter. These children are eager to talk; the therapist's sympathetic interest and attentiveness are all that is necessary. But for many children—to varying degrees, anxious, angry, or withdrawn—more active participation by the therapist is required. This aspect of the therapeutic process is generally referred to as establishing rapport with the child and then, a therapeutic alliance—some mutual understanding of the nature of the child's difficulties and some common purpose. And, of course, it is important, crucially important, to allay a child's initial anxieties and put him at ease. But more than rapport and more than establishing an alliance are involved in this process.

In my clinical experience, engagement with children is fostered by two essential therapeutic attitudes: (1) the therapist's empathic recognition of the child's distress (including the child's distress at being brought for treatment)—his worries, sadness, or disappointment, and perhaps particularly, his grievance—and (2) equally important, the therapist's enthusiastic, affirming responsiveness to the child's interests and positive affects. These attitudes—affirming responsiveness and empathic recognition of the child's distress or grievance—constitute our basic therapeutic stance with children. Clinical concepts derived from adult psychotherapy (e.g., abstinence, relative anonymity, and neutrality) have either limited relevance or are of secondary importance in the treatment of child patients. These processes of engagement are more than a preparatory phase of building rapport, more than a prelude to the real work of therapy; they are also processes of therapeutic change.

The importance of the therapist's enthusiastic, affirming responsiveness to the child's interests and positive affects is basic, perhaps even obvious. This aspect of child therapy, however, receives little explicit attention in most discussions of the therapeutic process and deserves more detailed consideration.

The therapeutic value of enhancing the child's positive affects is also insufficiently appreciated in recommendations for work with families.

Positive Affects: Theory and Research

There is now considerable research support for the importance of positive affects—in child development and throughout the life span. The role of positive emotions in optimal child development was the subject of an important review by Robert Emde (1991). Emde presents evidence for a "strong, separately organized, adaptive role for positive emotions in infancy" (p. 17). Of particular clinical relevance are research observations on positive affect sharing and caregiver availability.

Children are observed, toward the end of the first year of life, to look to a significant other and share a positive affect—to smile, for example, in the midst of an exploration or accomplishment. Emde refers to this behavior as "positive affect sharing." Osofsky (1995), in her studies of teenage mothers, reports the compelling observation that although positive affect sharing "occurs frequently in low-risk groups, adolescent mothers and their infants rarely show such activity" (p. 196).

Emde also cites the important contribution of positive affects to a caregiver's emotional availability. Emotional availability is enhanced by the caregiver's expressions of interest and pleasure in the child's ongoing activities. This is the conclusion, for example, from Sorce and Emde's (1981) "library" study: a mother's expressions of interest in her child's activities led to increased exploration and a higher developmental level of play. Emde notes, "If development is going well, we expect to see evidence of a range of emotions and a balance of interest and pleasure going back and forth between caregiver and child . . . when there are behavioral problems, it is characteristic for there to be little positive affect with a dampening of range in emotions." Emde suggests—and this point deserves particular emphasis—"In assessing problems in caregiver emotional availability, *a lack of positive emotions may be a more sensitive indicator of problems than an excess of negative emotions*" (pp. 15–16).

The importance of positive affects in normal child development, particularly moments of infant-caregiver mutual joy and delight, has been noted by many current developmental theorists. Demos (1984), for example, based on her observations of mother-child interactions, questioned "the implicit assumption in much psychiatric writing that in the absence of negative affect, positive affect will flourish unaided" (p. 25). Demos suggests that positive affects require "nurturance and support" and offers examples of how parents can encourage "the activity of wishing and the positive affects and fantasies associated with it," even while setting behavioral limits. Schore (1994), in his comprehensive review, has proposed that parent-infant interactions that generate high levels of shared interest and joyful affect directly influence "the experience-dependent growth of postnatally developing brain areas" (p. 391), particularly connections between limbic and cortical structures.

In recent years, the value of positive emotions for psychological and emotional health, not only in childhood, but throughout the lifespan, has also been increasingly recognized. The immediate adaptive function of negative emotions (e.g., fear or anger) is often obvious—these emotions trigger specific thought and action tendencies that enhance survival in response to environmental threats (Bonanno and Mayne, 2001). The survival value of positive emotions, however, is less readily apparent. Fredrickson (1998; Fredrickson and Branigan, 2001) has proposed a "broaden and build" theory of the adaptive value of positive emotions. Fredrickson argues that positive emotions have the general adaptive function of promoting exploration, creativity, and learning, and building social relationships that become resources in conditions of adversity. Fredrickson notes that positive emotions occur in the context to safety, rather than threat; and that whereas negative emotions *restrict* attention, positive emotions broaden our attentional focus. In this analysis, "as negative emotions are to threat, positive emotions are to opportunity" (Bonanno and Mayne, 2001, p. 401). Positive emotions restore flexible thinking that has been narrowed, for example, by anger or fear, and may serve as "effective antidotes for the lingering effects of negative emotions" (Fredrickson and Branigan, p. 135). Fredrickson and Branigan call this "the undoing effect." Fredrickson also reviews emerging experimental evidence, consistent with the clinical observations reported below, that positive emotions promote psychological resilience, trigger an "upward spiral" of mood, speed recovery from physiological distress, and promote coping with adversity, for example, bereavement.[1]

Interest and Positive Affect Sharing

Although the general trend of this research is compelling, the justification for my proposal regarding positive emotions in child therapy is based on clinical experience. The child therapist's responsiveness to the child's interests and positive emotions not only engages and sustains the child in the more difficult tasks of therapy, but appears to have considerable therapeutic value in its own right. If we are able to establish positive affect sharing with child patients (and, better yet, if we can help parents work through impediments to positive affect sharing in interactions with their children) we often observe substantial, early clinical improvement.

Young children, particularly, but adolescents also, are almost always willing—and usually eager—to share their interests; they often quite literally bring their interests to sessions.[2] The therapist's enthusiastic responsiveness to the child's interests engages the child; the child experiences our responsiveness as a form of "recognition" (Benjamin, 1988; 1995) or "appreciation" (Menaker, 2001). The child then looks to us for this kind of responsiveness and develops the expectation of an affirming response to his interests and positive affects. This expectation is already therapeutic. The child shows more enthusiasm and affective aliveness, both in and outside therapy sessions, less stubbornness and defiance in his interactions with parents and teachers, and recovers more quickly from negative affect states. In my experience, it is not uncommon for parents to report significant improvement early in treatment, when therapists may feel that they are still "just playing" with child patients and have not yet "done" anything. My clinical impression is that the enhancement of positive affects in child therapy seems to confer some degree of immunity to the child against the effects of emotional distress. These positive affective interactions, leading to the expectation of an affirming response, may operate as a protective factor in the emotional life of the child against the pathogenic forces of demoralization and rage.

This is a first function of children's play: the expansion of joyful affect. There are, of course, many other functions of play, including the learning and refinement of social skills, the socialization of aggression, and the expression and mastery of emotional conflict. What we observe most regularly in our interactions with children, however, is that children *enjoy* responsive play.[3] When a child finds in his therapist—and in his parents—an enthusiastic play partner, he responds with increased enthusiasm and affective aliveness.

We should therefore always ask, during our initial consultation with parents, about the child's interests or "passions." The information gleaned from this inquiry is often essential—both to our emerging understanding of the child's moods and behavior and as a guide in our initial efforts to facilitate engagement and dialogue.

And our first questions to children should also be about their interests—we ask the child about what he *likes*—and *likes to do*. In this way, we convey our interest in getting to know this child—what they like and don't like, what they want and don't want. Almost all children, except in moments of extreme sullenness or withdrawal, respond positively to our own genuine interest in learning about their interests. When we meet a child a second time, it is helpful to continue this discussion. We begin by saying, "I remember, you know a lot about space and science" or "You like the Yankees" or "You were telling me about..." The child is then likely to be less guarded in his answers when we begin to ask more difficult questions—if there are some things he might feel bad about, or times when he feels sad or angry, or if there is a problem we might be able to help with.

Floor Time

As a first illustration of the therapeutic potential of this mode of engagement, I have chosen an example from the work of Stanley Greeenspan. Greenspan and his colleagues (Greenspan and Wieder, 1997; 1998) have developed a program of therapeutic intervention for children with special needs that is of value to all child therapists. In a publication addressed to both lay and professional audiences (Greenspan, 1997), Greenspan describes his work with a 2-year-old autistic girl. I will quote extensively from Greenspan's report:

> This . . . girl neither spoke nor made any response to those around her, but would spend hours staring into space, rubbing persistently at a patch on the carpet. We saw in her abnormal repetition, however, not only a symptom of her autism, but a sign of *interest* and *motivation* (emphasis added)—at least involving that little spot of pile. Perhaps it could serve as an opening wedge for emotional connection and, later, learning. (p. 17)

This is a creative and enormously therapeutic insight—that the child's autistic symptoms were an expression of interest and motivation; that is, this little girl *liked* rubbing the carpet, she *wanted* to do this. This understanding is not apparent, certainly not self-evident, if we focus on the child's behavior as a symptom, a deficit in communication and social engagement. Continuing with Greenspan's report:

> We had the girl's mother place her hand next to hers, right on the favorite stretch of floor. The girl pushed it away, but the mother gently put it back. Again she pushed, again the hand returned. A cat and mouse game ensued and by the *third* day of this rudimentary interaction, the girl was *smiling* (emphasis added) while pushing her mother's hand away. From this tiny beginning grew an emotional connection, a relationship, and then thoughts and words. From pushing away an obstructing hand to seeking out that hand and then offering flirtatious grins and giggles, the child progressed to using gestures in a reciprocal non-verbal dialogue. When she began repeatedly flinging herself at her mother, the therapist recognized that this behavior gave her sensory pleasure. He instructed the mother to whinny like a horse each time her daughter lunged at her. Soon she was whinnying too, imitating her mother . . . Over time, mother and child pretended to be neighing horses, mooing cows, barking dogs . . . It wasn't long before stuffed bunnies were fighting and hugging . . . At age seven, this girl has a range of age-appropriate emotions, warm friendships and a lively imagination. She argues as well as her lawyer father, and scores in the low superior IQ range. (p. 17)

This is a dramatically successful and instructive treatment. Beginning with Greenspan's initial insight—that the child's behavior was a sign of interest—the mother's responses to the child's actions expand this sphere of the child's interest. At Greenspan's direction, the mother has taken the girl's autistic behavior and made a game out of it; through the mother's responses, the child is provided with the experience that her actions have an effect, an impact, on her mother. Excitement and joyful affect are created. A repetitive, solitary "interest" is transformed into pleasurable interaction; a solitary and stereotyped "game" becomes a more complex and open-ended game.

Greenspan has developed this therapeutic approach to autistic behavior into a highly successful treatment program he calls "Floor Time" (Greenspan and Wieder, 1997) and presents preliminary outcome data that compare favorably with behavioral treatments for autistic children (and perhaps even more favorably if the capacity for pleasure is included in outcome assessment measures). Greenspan (1993; 1995) has also presented the Floor Time program as a model for parent-child interactions, an aspect of "healthy parenting."

Greenspan's work with these children offers a paradigm for therapeutic engagement and change applicable to a wide range of children referred for consultation and treatment. From Greenspan's example, we can derive a basic principle of both therapeutic engagement and parent guidance: we *identify and respond to the child's expressions of interest* and then *expand the sphere of the child's interests*, helping the child develop increasingly confident expectations of adult responsiveness and then, increasingly complex interpersonal and emotional narratives. These interactions also promote the enhancement and refinement of social pragmatic skills that are intrinsic to interactive play.

It is important to note that, in this phase of treatment, our therapeutic goal is not to promote understanding; that is, our attention is focused not on the meaning of the child's play (for example, its symbolic or resistant aspects, as in classical psychoanalytic child therapy), but on our responsiveness to the affect and intention expressed in the child's playing. Our focus is on recognizing and sharing, with appropriately modulated enthusiasm, the child's initiative and interest, and their associated affects of excitement and enjoyment. In this way, we strengthen the child's sense of agency and what Fonagy and colleagues refer to as the "psychological self" (Fonagy, Moran, and Target, 1993), as the expectation of an affirming response becomes a part of the child's inner world, or psychic reality.

The principle of joyful, affirming responsiveness is a first principle of child development and a first—among many—parental functions. In normal development, the child's expectation of an affirming response, beginning with the parents' joyful and prideful delight in each developmental milestone—the child's first smiles and words and succeeding achievements in cognitive, social, and athletic competence—has an important role in sustaining the child (as all of us are sustained throughout life) in the face of the inevitable frustrations, disappointments, and disillusionments of growing up, life's many small defeats and crises of demoralization.

* * *

The following brief clinical examples of engagement with withdrawn and anxious children, taken from my own practice, are offered as encouragement, especially for beginning child therapists, to adopt a responsive, playful way of being with child patients.

Alan

Alan is an 8-year-old boy, referred for therapy because of difficulty establishing peer relationships. Alan is unable to engage in group activities with other children. If allowed, he would spend all weekend playing video games or watching television. Alan has few friends his own age and he is rarely invited to birthday parties. He often ignores other children when they approach him to play, or he may abruptly turn away. When playing one-to-one with another child, Alan's interest quickly wanes as soon as the child wants to play "their way." Other children have called Alan a "baby."

Mr. and Mrs. C. also report significant problems of attention span and distractibility. In school, Alan seems to be doing well in his reading and math skills; however, his teachers describe him as restless, fidgety, and needing frequent redirection to tasks. Alan is also afraid to be alone in some rooms of his house.

Like many children referred for evaluation and treatment, these presenting problems suggest a complex developmental disorder, requiring comprehensive evaluation. Evaluations when Alan was in preschool noted unusual sensory sensitivities and delays in Alan's language and motor skills.

When I met Alan in the waiting room, he was sitting, curled up against his mother, holding a toy ray-gun.

"Hi Alan"

Initially, Alan ignored me.

I greeted him again.

Alan aimed his ray-gun at me and pretended to shoot.

I noticed, in this action, a faint smile, and I took a chance. I ducked Alan's ray, took cover, pointed my finger, and shot back, "Pssh."

Now, Alan smiled broadly. He took his gun and shot again; this time, he "got me."

"Hey," I asked, noticing the action figures Alan was holding, "Is that Buzz Lightyear? And who is that guy?" Alan then began to tell me—with enthusiasm—about the action figures he had brought with him for us to play with. The next week he brought others, and then others—and we were now friends. Gradually, Alan began to tell me about his worries, especially about being teased and laughed at by his peers.

In Alan's development, we note a common pathogenic cycle—a pathway that begins with Alan's intrinsic difficulties in social engagement and his anxiety in peer group interactions, and then continues—with increasing ostracism by peers, withdrawal into fantasy, and failure to develop social skills. We begin to ameliorate these difficulties through interactive play. From this beginning, the therapeutic process then fosters the development of more mature social relationships—Alan's ability to engage with others, to share interests, to express his own needs, and to take into account the needs of others.

John: "Star Wars" and Checkers

John is an intelligent 8-year-old boy, whose parents expressed concern about his frequent temper tantrums and uncooperativeness at home and his disregard of personal hygiene. Mr. and Mrs. S. also observed, somewhat as an afterthought, that John often seemed unhappy. To his teachers, however, John's unhappiness was palpable. In school, John was aloof and "reclusive"; he rarely spoke to other children, except for his one friend; he did not participate in any sports or games, or in academic projects that required either imagination or collaboration with other students; and on at least one occasion he had alarmed his teachers with vague references to "shooting" while standing apart from his classmates on the playing field.

When I met John, he was standing, cowering, in the corner of my waiting room, while his two younger siblings played on the floor with blocks. He told me, in this first meeting, echoing his mother's complaints, that he had two problems—procrastination and "wasting time." Soon, however, John began to talk about his interest in the Stars Wars saga and the Star Wars computer games that occupied all of John's free time. With this exception, I found John singularly lacking in joyfulness or enthusiasm; nor could I detect any joyfulness in the lives of his parents. Mr. and Mrs. S. seemed largely unaware of the sadness and loneliness, and perhaps also retaliatory fantasies, that increasingly dominated John's emotional life. Mrs. S. thought John was often "manipulative" and asked, each week, if I would talk with John about being more cooperative, or nicer to his siblings. I, of course, had little interest in this approach, and, in any case, John offered only polite, perfunctory answers to my often perfunctory questions. Mr. S., whom I met with infrequently, appeared serious and reserved, but interested in what I had to say. He seemed to regard my recommendation that he spend some time each evening playing with John, especially the Star Wars computer games John enjoyed and knew so much about, as a novel, but intriguing, idea. (I had asked John if he played these games with his father; John looked puzzled, "No," he answered, "He has his *own* computer.") The effect of this simple suggestion, however, was quite dramatic. John's mood brightened; he began to do his homework immediately after school, "so I can have time to play with my dad." Sadly, Mr. S. was unable to sustain this involvement with his son.

For many months, John spoke very little about any problem or troubling feeling. But, with increasing enthusiasm, and then increasing imagination, John talked to me about his detailed knowledge of Star Wars, as we played checkers; and there was nothing perfunctory about John's engagement in this talk and play. John eagerly looked forward to his sessions; he remembered each week's game; and he was exquisitely sensitive to any momentary distraction or inattention on my part. I allowed John to win these games, and after each defeat, John instructed me on his selection of the winning strategy and I spoke to John appreciatively about his tactics and skill. Soon, the games became more inventive and expansive: checker pieces became Star Wars characters and John took greater and greater gleeful pleasure, as younger children ordinarily do, in his victories—and my ineptitude. John then began to laugh, at first furtively, then more openly—at my mistakes and I quietly welcomed this increased affective aliveness.

All of this, of course—John's increasing animation, his enthusiastic sharing of knowledge, and his avoidance of experiences that were too painful to talk about—is perhaps unremarkable, typical of the initial phase of engagement in any child treatment, unusual only in the degree of John's affective constriction, a cardinal symptom of the pathological development I have attempted to describe.

After almost a year of treatment, John began to talk about feelings; at first tentatively, then with poignancy and directness, beginning, belatedly, a second phase of therapy. John told me, first, that he was "a little nervous" about beginning fourth grade. I made note of this simple comment as the first I could recall in which John had spoken directly of *any* affect. Later, John began to speak of the injuries and painful affects he experienced daily in his peer relationships ("I don't fit in," John told me; "I don't even know what this World Series thing is"). In these discussions, John spoke with some defensiveness ("I'm basically an independent person," John told me). But he also showed surprising insight and empathy for other children and an introspective capacity that I suspect had always been present, but too painful for John to talk about, qualities entirely hidden throughout almost two years of treatment.

By this time, John was a happier child; he made new friends and found more pleasure in all his activities, private and social. There were, of course, still significant difficulties in John's adjustment—avoidances and inhibitions, resentment, envy, and defiant attitudes. As happens frequently, however, John's parents, although now appreciative of his improvement, were satisfied with his progress and ready to terminate John's treatment well before either John or I were, a premature termination I was only briefly able to forestall.

Being Heard

The enhancement of positive affects, however, despite its importance in both normal development and child treatment, represents only one dimension of a complex, multidimensional, therapeutic process. As a complement to the enhancement of positive affects, the therapist's empathic recognition of the child's painful emotions, particularly the child's *grievance*, presents a second opportunity for therapeutic engagement. When we are able to identify the sources of a child's distress or grievance (and help parents understand and listen, if not empathically, at least less critically, to their child's grievance) we initiate an essential process of therapeutic change: the development of increased tolerance for distressing affects, more successful recovery from emotional injuries, and a more stable sense of self.

The essence of this process has been described by Bach (1994), in a deceptively simple formulation, as "being heard."[4] Children who are chronically "not heard" are likely to become increasingly defiant or demoralized. We all know, of course, the experience of not being heard—we become angry; our voices get louder, more insistent, and more certain; we may exaggerate or become stubborn, even self-righteous. This is true for all of us, children certainly no less than adults. When a child's protests continue to be unrecognized, or met with hostility, his *distress* will now be expressed as a *grievance*—what began as a *need* has now become a self-righteous *demand*. Chronic grievance is a particularly malignant process, marked by increasingly intractable and "impenitent" attitudes (Spillius, 1997).

Having allayed, at least to some extent, the child's initial anxiety and established our noncritical interest in getting to know this child, and having created some playfulness and positive affect sharing, we can now begin to ask the child if there is something he might want to talk about—perhaps a problem he may be having, in his family, at school, or with his friends, something the child might "feel bad" about. And we briefly explain what most children already know—that this is our job, to help kids and families with their "bad feelings."

In response to these tactful inquiries, many children will identify a grievance. The child may tell us—tentatively and cautiously, or at other times, vehemently and repetitively—what he feels is "not fair." His teachers are too strict or "mean"; or his parents "always" yell at him or punish him (and they do not punish his siblings). He may tell us what he is not allowed to do, that he is not given any freedom; or about social cliques at school and being "left out"; that he is blamed for everything; that his parents are "always angry"; and, perhaps especially, that "no one listens" to him. Without taking at face value everything that children tell us, it is still instructive how frequently children complain that no one listens to them.

Parents of course, also have grievances. They are often certain that they are "right" and that the child must change; if they are critical, it is because, "he has to learn..." These are complex and difficult clinical problems; to solve them, we will need to understand the legitimate concerns of both parents and children. Most often, we will agree with the parents' goals, but suggest a different means of getting there.

In childhood, a failure of being heard is likely to set in motion a vicious cycle of pathogenic events: as the child's grievance is more often expressed in some form of defiance and retaliation (often against siblings) or as an unreasonable demand, his behavior elicits increasingly critical and punitive responses from parents (and teachers) and a family atmosphere is now dominated by criticism and argument. Parents are less able to "hear" the child's distress; instead, they hear only the unreasonable quality of the child's refusal or "overreaction." These angry, critical, and inflexible parent-child dialogues then inhibit the development of social maturity—the child's ability to compromise and to take into account the legitimate needs of others.

Being heard arrests these potentially malignant intrapsychic and interpersonal processes. The therapeutic benefit of this form of recognition is, arguably, greater for children than for adults, before pathological attitudes have been firmly established (and then resolutely defended).

In these initial conversations with children, we begin with some effort to understand the child's point of view. Often, this is not difficult. We readily understand, for example, "how bad kids feel when parents are angry at them a lot... or at each other... and when kids get put in the middle..." But it is not always easy—for parents or therapists—to hear a defiant child (or a cynical adolescent). The child's stated grievance, perhaps especially when expressed as an insistent demand for "things," often masks a deeper unhappiness that he cannot yet talk about. And, of course, what the child tells us may not be the whole story.

At times, in spite of our empathic intent, we may be taken aback by the vehemence of the child's complaints, his apparent lack of empathy ("My problem is my sister... she's a moron..."), or the unyielding nature of his blaming and denial. The more insistently a child blames others, the more likely that he feels chronically "not heard." Often, these children have come to expect criticism and blame. Listening has been replaced by argument, and defensiveness and denial have become firmly established. In these cases, we may decide, in order to arrest this vicious cycle of events, to begin the therapeutic process with extended parent counseling sessions.

Children, however, are not always as demanding and unreasonable as they sometimes seem to be. The child knows that he cannot get everything he wants and that his parents should not give in to all of his demands. And although children may repeatedly blame others, they do not always believe everything they say. All children (and most adolescents), except in the midst of an ongoing argument, acknowledge the need for rules and limits. It is commonly said that defiant children are "asking for limits" and there is, perhaps, some truth in this formulation. More fundamentally, however, these children are asking to be heard; and they are willing, when their legitimate needs and concerns have been acknowledged, to accept some limit on their demands.

Our task of understanding a child's grievance is also made easier when we realize that the child has almost always made some effort in the direction of accommodating his parents' requests. This effort, however, has often gone unnoticed (or is "not enough"), hardening the child's grievance. When we are able to recognize and appreciate (and, again, help parents appreciate) these small efforts on the part of the child, we begin to unlock a stubborn impasse between parents and children. If we are able to listen patiently, it is likely that the child has identified one link in a sequence, or vicious cycle, of events that we can help both the child and his parents understand. Children do not expect us to agree, but to listen.

Sharings

For many child therapists, the injunction against therapist self-disclosure, with its long and important history, has become almost a cardinal rule.

There are good reasons, in work with adult patients, for therapists to be cautious about overt self-disclosures—to protect the integrity of the therapeutic process and to protect the patient from the therapist's excessive zeal. Freud (1912) warned strongly against the use of the analyst's personal influence in psychoanalytic therapy and he accepted this restriction of the analyst's role as one of the inherent limitations of psychoanalytic treatment. His admonitions have become part of the generally accepted framework of psychotherapy, with both children and adults.

But children are different, and clinical work with children suffers when we impose on our child patients a model of treatment derived from psychotherapy with adults. Most experienced child therapists accept these differences and accommodate their style of engaging and communicating to the needs and anxieties of their child patients. Still, in a recent survey of experienced child therapists—of different theoretical orientations (Capobianco and Farber, 2005)—only a small minority of respondents reported the use of self-disclosure in their work with child patients, and an even smaller number believed that self-disclosures "advanced treatment aims."[5]

My own clinical experience has taught a different lesson. To promote engagement with anxious children, I often speak openly about myself, almost from the first moment I am introduced to a child or as soon as the child has indicated an interest—perhaps in a book they have been reading in the waiting room, a video game, a musical instrument, or a baseball team. I ask children about their interest and tell them some of what I know about it, or what I don't know, so that they can teach me. Most children, who have not been taught the technical rules and injunctions of psychotherapy, seem surprised and even delighted by these small sharings of ourselves and almost universally experience these discussions not as intrusions, but as evidence of our interest.[6] These statements convey to the child an atmosphere of normalcy and openness (as opposed to the scrutiny and criticism he fears), and foster the child's openness in talking to us. Along with our empathic understanding and enthusiastic interest, talking personally to children establishes the therapist as a noncritical and nonthreatening presence and promotes the positive affective interactions that are a sine qua non of effective psychotherapy with children. I have come to regard these small, normalizing, self-disclosures, including the therapist's expression of affect in the course of play, as helpful in the engagement of most children, necessary in the engagement of some. In contrast, a less participatory, more "observing" mode of relating to children, even a friendly, interested, observing stance, is experienced by many children as alien, and they respond with some form of resistance, open or covert. My recommendation, therefore, to beginning child therapists, who have often borrowed for work with children a model or style of relating developed to facilitate communication (and the expression of transference) with adult patients, is to relax with child patients—to be animated and playful, at times even silly, and to be thoughtful, but not shy, in talking about yourself.

Therapeutic work with children also needs to take into account a simple, readily verifiable, clinical fact: when we talk about ourselves to children, children listen attentively and they remember what we say. Many years ago, I was concluding the successful treatment of Carl, an intelligent and creative but anxious 9-year-old boy, whose presenting problems had included an unusual phobia. In addition to many common fears and avoidances, Carl was unable to watch some films shown in his third grade classroom or even to read passages from some children's books. Carl tried, over the course of several weeks, to overcome this phobic reaction by reading a few pages at a time, each week, in his sessions with me. The therapy had, in my mind, focused on the analysis of these symptoms and also Carl's dreams. Because of my interest in the mechanisms of therapeutic change with child patients, I asked Carl, as we were ending treatment, what he remembered of all the things we had talked about. He replied, without any hesitation, and with evident pleasure, "I know all the things you stink at."[7]

More often than not, children should look forward to, and smile in, their therapy sessions. In my consultative and supervisory experience, the therapist's effort to create, or renew, a more playful, responsive engagement with her child patients, including the judicious use of therapist self-disclosures, often revitalizes a stagnant therapy, overburdened by an excess of inquiry, interpretation, or problem-solving. And it is in this context—of enthusiastic and playful engagement—that we are able to most successfully challenge or "nudge" children (Fonagy and Target, 1998) toward more mature relatedness and help them accept painful or disagreeable affects. The masters of child therapy, regardless of theory, intuitively know this. The case reports of gifted child therapists are remarkable for their humor, playfulness, and modesty, guided by the therapist's empathy for the joys and enthusiasms, as well as the anxieties, of childhood.

Notes

1. Fredrickson also presents an experimental result with direct relevance to the psychotherapeutic situation: subjects who were first presented with an affirming experience showed greater willingness, at a later time, to accept or consider negative information (1998, p. 319).

   Izard and Ackerman (2000) present a similar analysis of the adaptive function of positive emotions in their discussion of the emotion of joy. "Joy strengthens social bonds, especially parent-child bonds that are essential to survival, promotes affiliative behavior and heightens openness to experience." Izard and Ackerman also suggest that joy has "recuperative powers that can serve as an antidote to distress" and cite Lazarus and his colleagues' view that "positive emotions function as breathers in relieving stress and sustain coping in taxing situations" (p. 258). In his review, Emde (1991) also suggests that positive emotions may serve as a "buffer" in times of stress.

2. Spiegel (1996), in an excellent presentation of an Interpersonal approach to child therapy, recommends that child therapists discourage children from bringing their own toys to sessions, in order to facilitate a discussion with the child of his motivations for bringing his toys ("as a way of diverting the therapy, to display their skills . . . or . . . to enable them to brag about their possessions," p. 125). I disagree. In my experience, there is no disadvantage to allowing, even encouraging, a child to bring to his therapy sessions whatever he wants to share with us. Bringing his toys (or cards, dolls, or music) facilitates engagement; and the child's feelings and motivations, including his avoidances, can always be discussed.
3. Panksepp (1998) begins his discussion of the neuroscience of play with the commonplace, but important, observation that, "When children are asked what they like to do more than anything else, the most common answer is 'to play!' " (p. 280).
4. Bach describes his work with a young adult anorexic patient who needed to find in her analysis "some personal psychic space in which her own volition, effectance, and continuity could be vitally experienced. *This space . . . in healthy people is created . . . when they speak and expect to be heard*" (p. 157, emphasis added).
5. In this survey, psychoanalytic/psychodynamic therapists were somewhat less likely than cognitive/cognitive-behavioral or eclectic therapists to make use of self-disclosure with child patients. Capobianco and Farber acknowledge some limitations to their conclusions. The low frequency of therapist self-disclosures may, to some extent, have been a function of the restricted content of the survey; therapists were asked, for example, only about self-disclosures in their answers to questions asked by child patients and about disclosures of facts rather than feelings or personal reactions.
6. There are, however, some important exceptions to this statement, for example, children who are unusually sullen or suspicious.
7. Self-disclosures by child therapists also serve, at appropriate times, a second important therapeutic function. At moments of acute distress, many children derive immediate, visible emotional support—and, one hopes, some lasting increment of self-acceptance—from the child therapist's generative, humanizing, self-disclosures. I have discussed this dimension of child and adolescent therapy in a previous article (Barish, 2004).

7

Empathy

The importance of the therapist's empathy is universally acknowledged, at least as an essential precondition, for all effective psychotherapy, including psychotherapy with children and families. In recent years, however, clinical and theoretical interest in empathy—with some exceptions (see, especially, Bromfield, 2007; Greene and Ablon, 2006)—appears to have waned, and this trend is particularly apparent in writing about children. The concept of empathy is regarded by many as vague, unscientific, and subject to frequent misuse. Contemporary psychoanalytic child therapists have focused attention on processes related to empathy (for example, mentalization and reflective functioning, Fongay and Target, 1998; Fongay et al., 2002) recognition and intersubjectivity, Frankel, 1998; or insightfulness, Koren-Karie, Oppenheim, and Goldsmith, 2007 but tend to eschew empathy as an organizing theoretical concept. Empathy also plays a small role in the theory and technique of cognitive and behavioral approaches to child therapy.[1]

I believe this trend is unfortunate. The art of empathic listening remains our most fundamental clinical skill, and, in my opinion, our most effective therapeutic "technique." In this chapter, I will present a perspective on the nature of empathy that highlights the intrinsic relationship of empathy and affect. I will then consider how the child therapist's empathy is expressed and how the experience of empathic understanding is beneficial in the emotional life of the child, and I will offer a specific hypothesis on the therapeutic efficacy of empathic understanding in clinical work with children.

The Nature of Empathy

It may be helpful to briefly review some classic and contemporary views on the definition and nature of empathy. In both everyday usage and in clinical practice, empathy is understood as a distinctive emotional-cognitive attitude towards others—an attitude, or process, in which we make some effort to put aside our own perspective and needs in order to understand the subjective experience of another person. The empathic attitude is characterized, especially, by a conscious effort to suspend criticism or judgment. Eisenberg (2000), who provides an excellent concise review, defines empathy as "an affective response that stems from the apprehension or comprehension of another's emotional state or condition, and that is identical or very similar to what the other person is feeling or would be expected to feel." (p. 677). Eisenberg adds, as do many others, in order to distinguish empathy from emotional contagion, that, "empathy requires at least some differentiation of one's own and another's emotional state or condition." Very young infants, therefore, Eisenberg notes, experience emotional contagion, but not empathy.

Freud, with characteristic incisiveness, wrote that empathy is "the mechanism by means of which we are enabled to take up any attitude at all toward another mental life" (1921, p. 110). Kohut understood empathy in a similar sense. In an early essay, Kohut (1959) defined empathy as a *mode of observation* (not, it is important to note, as a therapeutic technique or a bond between people) through which we learn about another person's psychological life. In this most important sense, it is only through empathy that our perception or understanding becomes *psychological.* "We designate phenomena as mental, psychic, or psychological if our mode of observation includes introspection and empathy *as an essential constituent*... A phenomenon is 'somatic', 'behavioristic', or 'social' if our methods of observation do not predominantly include introspection and empathy" (pp. 208–209). Somewhat later, Kohut (1971) refined this understanding and defined empathy as "a mode of cognition which is specifically attuned to the perception of complex psychological configurations" (p. 300). It was only in his final writings (1982) that Kohut wrote about empathy in a second, perhaps more familiar, sense, that is, the therapeutic or sustaining power of empathy.

Carl Rogers (cited in Eisenberg) defined therapeutic empathy as the therapist's effort "to perceive the internal frame of reference of another with accuracy and with the emotional components and meanings which pertain thereto..." and later added, "nonjudgmentally understanding and communicating one's understanding to another... checking with him/her as to the accuracy of your sensings, and being guided by the responses you receive" (p. 677). Rogers includes, in this statement, not only empathic understanding, but also empathic communication. Rogers' emphasis on being guided by empathy will be especially important in understanding the role of empathy in the treatment of children.

More recently, Baron-Cohen (2003), in the context of a much more controversial thesis (i.e., the "essential difference" between male and female brains) has argued that empathy is a fundamental mode of cognition—of perception, information processing, and imagination—that has evolved for the perception of *affect.* Baron-Cohen suggests that empathy co-evolved with primate parental investment and the consequent need for mothers to perceive infant expressions of distress. He notes that empathic cognition is *required* for the perception of affect—and not required for processing non-affective information. In contrast to Freud and Kohut, however, Baron-Cohen believes that empathic *cognition* is inseparable from the *behavioral* responses of concern and caring.

Baron-Cohen distinguishes *empathic* cognition from what he calls *systemizing* cognition. Systemizing thought (in Baron-Cohen's view, the characteristic mode of cognition of the male brain) is "the drive to build and understand systems, including logical, scientific, and mathematical thought, broadly understood" (p. 3). Systemizing cognition attempts to construct predictable, logical relationships; to understand the rules that govern the behavior of objects; to figure out "how things work." Emotions, however, can rarely be understood in this way—the inputs we need to understand emotions (for example, facial and vocal expressiveness) are too simultaneous and too complex to be efficiently processed by the systemizing mode of thought.

Bloom (2004) has offered an even more general formulation: that we engage in empathic cognition when we regard others as having *purposes* or *intentions*. And the recent discovery of "mirror" neurons in higher primates and humans (Gallese, 2001)—neurons that fire both when we perform an action and when we observe others performing the same action—provides a significant advance in our understanding of a neural substrate of empathy, especially our ability to perceive *intention* in others.[2] Empathic behaviors have been observed in some non-human primates and, perhaps, in other mammals as well. The primatologist Frans DeWaal (2001) reports that, "chimpanzees will approach a victim of attack, put an arm around her and gently pat her back, or groom her. These reassuring encounters, termed *consolations*, are so predictable that my students and I have recorded hundreds of instances" (p. 326). DeWaal adds that, in contrast to chimpanzees, "In monkeys, consolation has never been demonstrated. On the contrary, monkeys often avoid victims of aggression."[3] These discoveries and observations have important implications for our understanding of neurological disorders characterized by deficits in empathic capacity and, potentially, for the origins of language (Rizzolatti and Arbib, 1998) and morality—"what makes us human" (Bloom, 2004). But they do not yet provide a clinical, or therapeutic, theory of empathy.[4]

Demos (1984), in an important discussion of the relationship between empathy and affect based on her observations of infant—caregiver interactions, presents a useful paradigm for empathic understanding and communication that brings us closer to a clinical model for the expression of empathy in the therapeutic process with children and families. Consistent with recent advances in the theory of emotions, Demos identifies three components of affective experience: (1) "the triggering event or stimulus" (now commonly referred to as an appraisal), (2) "the affective experience per se," and (3) "the response of the organism to its own affective experience, which involves the recruitment in memory of past experiences, as well as motor responses and plans" (p. 11). In Demos' model, optimal empathic communications attempt to convey—in words or in actions—an understanding of all three components of the child's affective experience; for example, that the child is in distress, what evoked her distress (what the child is upset "about"), and the child's plans or goals—what the child is attempting to do to alleviate her distress.

Demos offers the everyday example of a mother who notices that her child is looking at—and beginning to reach for—a pair of scissors. From the child's point of view, this is a situation of *interest* and exploration; from the parent's point view, it is a situation of danger. Many common parent-child interactions share this structure—the child wants to play and explore; the parent needs to protect the child from harm. Demos notes that when a parent is able to recognize in this situation, not only the danger, but also the child's interest, this empathic appreciation opens up opportunities for the parent to respond in a way that insures the child's safety but does not entirely thwart her exploration (for example, by providing the child a safer toy to play with).[5]

Before discussing the role of empathy in the therapeutic process with children, I need to note several additional, essential characteristics of empathy:

(1) When we listen and communicate in the empathic mode, we convey, in some form, a non-judgmental appreciation of the child's *affects* and *intentions—not*, in that moment, the child's *behavior* and its *consequences.*

(2) Clinical empathy involves the therapist's effort to appreciate *what is important to the child,* especially those aspects of the child's experience that have not yet—from the child's point of view—been sufficiently acknowledged or understood.[6]

(3) When our responses are influenced by empathic resonance or empathic understanding, we alter our behavior, sometimes in subtle ways and often outside our awareness, in response to the subjective state of the other person—that is, we allow the other person to *influence* us. Many common expressions of empathy in everyday interactions are of this kind, for example, when we slow down the pace of our speech or alter our inflection and our vocabulary in speaking to children (or to others who are less fluent in our language). These subtle accommodations probably contribute to our feeling of connection or comfort with others, perhaps a beginning form of "intersubjective relatedness." And many common parental (and marital) *failures* of empathy are of this kind. The absence of subtle empathic accommodations to others is jarring in everyday interactions and profoundly destructive in close interpersonal relationships. It is often highly disturbing to hear adults talk to children without making these adjustments; when, for example, a parent knows that a child is angry or upset, but (because the parent disapproves of the child's behavior) the parent remains unmoved.[7]

(4) Finally, empathy acts as an instinctive inhibitory mechanism on aggression, on the inclination to cause injury or harm (Feshbach, 1989). We have known this, of course, for a long time—that it is far easier to act aggressively and to cause injury to someone who has been dehumanized, who is

"other" or not *like us*, for example, to shoot a "target" from a distance, in this way, reducing our instinctive empathic resonance, rather than a "person" who can be seen.

How Is Empathy Expressed in Clinical Work with Children?

To briefly review: Empathy is a mode of cognition that enables us to perceive affect and intention in others. Empathy, however, is not only a mode of cognition, but at the same time, an emotion; and, like all emotions, empathy has a characteristic action disposition: to provide an affirming or solacing response. An empathic response consists of any behavior—even a subtle alteration of our posture or vocal inflection—that communicates an appreciation of the child's emotions and attempts to either prolong the child's positive feeling or mitigate her distress.

If we consider empathy broadly, in this way, it becomes evident that the child therapist's empathy is deeply intrinsic and continuously present in our interactions with children—to a great extent, empathy guides the entire therapeutic process. The child therapist's empathy is expressed (1) in our consistent attention to the child's affects and intentions and in our effort to understand events in the life of child from the child's point of view. We are not—at that moment—concerned with the consequences of the child's behavior; (2) in our appreciation of *what is important to the child*; (3) in subtle alterations of *our* behavior, for example, our vocal tone and inflection, in response to the child's distinctive affective style; (4) in our appreciation of the child's positive emotions; for example, the child's excitement and attachment to a new or favorite doll or toy, their passion for collecting, their love of animals, or their pride in new developmental achievements—how fast they can run, how far they can throw, or how well they have learned to read, or draw, or build; and (5) in our effort not to cause further injury to the child, especially injury to the child's self-esteem.

The child therapist's expressions of empathy begin before we have met the child, when we talk with parents—as we should in every initial consultation—about how the child is likely to feel about being brought to our office and how parents might best talk with her about this. Our empathic responsiveness continues when we encounter the child in our waiting room and make note of—and in some way acknowledge—her anxiety or her tentative expressions of curiosity and eagerness. Among our first, and most basic, expressions of empathy is our genuine, appropriately modulated, but still enthusiastic expressions of interest in the child's interests—what the child likes and wants—to which almost all children respond with increased communication and affective aliveness.

Our empathy is also continuously present when we respond to the child's changing expressions of affect in the course of a session, whether these are expressions of anxiety and distress, or excitement and pride, or gleeful triumph; in our understanding of the child's conflicts, defenses, and resistances; and in our ongoing assessments of the child's receptivity—verbal and non-verbal—to what we say. In this model, even not speaking—knowing when to be silent—can be an empathic response, for example, when a child says, "I don't want to talk about it."

For beginning child therapists, I would offer some specific advice: when we communicate empathically with children, we speak—and act—with animation and with our own affective expressiveness. We should use adjectives, qualifiers, and gestures; we should talk to children, for example, about what they *really, really* want; or that they *really* didn't want to go to school, or come to therapy today. Or, when we talk with children who (perhaps because of emotional conflict) are uncomfortable with the experience of intense affect, we suggest that perhaps they were *kind of* nervous or *kind of* mad; or that they sometimes might feel *a little* mad, but they don't really *like* to feel mad. It is only in this way that we communicate our empathic understanding of *this* child—the child's unique, complex emotional experience.

The Therapeutic Function of Empathy

We can now more fully appreciate the therapeutic function of empathy—both in the clinical situation and in optimal child development. I have proposed that the psychopathology of childhood and adolescence, whether expressed as a disturbance of mood or behavior, results from the persistence of negative emotions—and the complex transformations of these emotions—in the mind of the child. In this model, the critical factor determining the psychological health of the developing child—and the central goal of our therapeutic efforts—is the development of emotional resilience or psychological immunity—the child's ability to bounce back from the inevitable disappointments, sadness, frustration, and anger of childhood. In healthy emotional development, reparative processes function to heal emotional injuries—to restore in the child a positive sense of herself and her future, some form of positive expectation. In my opinion, the essential component of these reparative experiences is *empathy*.

I would therefore offer a specific hypothesis regarding the therapeutic function of empathy in clinical work with children: each accurate empathic communication, especially our empathic recognition of the child's distress and grievance, *arrests the spread of potentially malignant psychological events in the mind of the child*. In this way, empathic understanding promotes a decisive change in the child's attitudes and behavior, and in her inner world of affect and fantasy.

Consider this process in more detail. Empathic responsiveness to the child's *positive* emotions enhances the child's experience of these emotions. A developmental pathway has been strengthened—a pathway that begins with the child's expressions of interest and leads to excitement and to joy. These experiences strengthen the child's expectation of an affirming response; both the child and her parents will look forward to opportunities to continue these interactions.[8]

Empathic understanding of the child's distress or grievance reduces the emotional arousal associated with these affects. Again, in my view, prolonged arousal of negative emotions, including their cognitive, physiological, and behavioral components—their elaboration in the child's fantasy, attitudes, and behavior—is the primary pathogenic process in childhood. In moments of empathic understanding, as we all know from personal experience, anger subsides, and sadness and shame are attenuated. Each accurate communication of empathic understanding also creates some increment of hopefulness and some diminution of the qualities of urgency and inflexibility that are characteristic of pathological emotional states.

Empathic understanding therefore promotes reduced stress at the physiological level and increased flexibility at the cognitive—emotional level. Behaviorally, we see less withdrawal, less defiance, and less argument. Expressions of empathy also promote initiative (as opposed to stubbornness and refusal) and an explicit or implicit future orientation, essential components of a resilient self. Experiences of empathic understanding then allow maturing processes to take place—the child becomes, in small increments, more open to educative and socializing influences, to compromise and active problem-solving. In this way, empathic understanding facilitates a fulcrum shift in emotional development—away from urgent and insistent demands and toward tolerance for disappointments and frustrations, and acceptance of personal responsibility.

This perspective on the beneficial effects of empathy in child development reminds us of what we should already know well—that children will more willingly and openly listen to us when they feel that we have listened to them, when we have understood their legitimate needs and concerns—a basic principle of all dialogue (Yankelovich, 1999)—between couples, between parents and their children, and between groups and nations. In my experience, when we are able to communicate empathic understanding to children—and, especially, when we are able to promote improved empathic understanding between parents and their children—we have achieved a significant therapeutic result, more profound and more lasting, I would propose, than we are able to achieve in any other way.

Difficulties and Limitations

This is a profoundly therapeutic effect. But is it always possible? And is it enough? To remain empathic—noncritical and nonjudgmental—in the midst of a child's angry protest or stubborn refusal, both for therapists and especially for parents, is hardly an easy task. How can we remain empathic when the child denies any bad feelings, refuses to cooperate with basic tasks, or acts in a hurtful or dangerously aggressive manner in response to minimal provocation? Or when the child tells us that it's everyone else's fault; that she didn't do anything wrong, and she should not have been punished? And is an *empathic* response always the *right* response?

In my opinion, this difficult empathic effort on the part of the child therapist remains our most distinctive contribution to the emotional development and well-being of the child. Our effort to remain empathic is what *makes us therapists*—and what is healing to children. If we listen patiently to the child's grievance, we will often find some truth in "her side" of the story, some previously unnoticed provocation or hurt feeling. Often, we will learn that she has made some effort at compliance and cooperation that has not yet been recognized. Again, it is helpful to recall that, more often than not, the child knows that her demands are unreasonable and even that some punishment is called for. She is stuck, however, in some form of argument, justifying her actions. She has already heard criticism and been given advice; now, she wants her parents to "just listen," so that she can let go of the argument. And no matter how adamant or vociferous her defense ("He started it"), arguing with her will, in all likelihood, just make her better at arguing—more defiant in her attitudes and more stubborn in her self-defense. The more extensive this process has become, the more difficult our therapeutic task—and the more patience will be required.

But empathy is not enough. Children, no less than adults, do not readily let go of habitual defenses and resistances. In most instances, therefore, successful treatment of children requires a second phase of therapy: we need to challenge children—still guided by our understanding of the child's emotions and still within a context of empathic understanding—to think or act differently, perhaps in ways they had not thought of, or have refused to do.

There is another important limitation to the role of empathy, both in development and, to some extent, in the therapeutic situation. The developmental principle of empathic responsiveness is complemented by a second principle: the parent's socializing function. Every family—and every society—has the task of socializing its children. Parents accept this socializing role as a primary parental responsibility—to educate their children, in the broad sense—to foster the skills and moral values necessary for their survival and the survival of their primary social group. There are many situations—especially situations of safety and those involving the rights of others, and when it is essential to get things done—when empathic responses are not the right responses and the child's feelings do not count. In these instances, what matters *is* the child's behavior and its consequences. Children, early in childhood, come to understand this; and for all of us, throughout life, recognizing the limits of empathy is an essential aspect of emotional maturity. The child comes to know that she must put aside her own needs and feelings; that, at this moment, what matters are the needs of others.

We can therefore distinguish two developmental principles and two kinds of parental responses: (1) empathic responses, that attenuate the child's distress and strengthen her sense of agency and confidence, and (2) socializing responses, that help children recognize the rights of others and develop an internalized sense of rules and law, of discipline and restraint. In the chapters that follow, I will discuss these dimensions of development and of the therapeutic process.

Sara: "It's Not Worth It"

Sara is a 13-year-old girl, the oldest of four siblings in a family of considerable intellectual achievement. For several years, Sara's lack of interest and motivation, especially with respect to academic work, had been of great concern to her parents; during the past school year, her academic performance deteriorated significantly. A recent neuropsychological evaluation confirmed Sara's excellent verbal and non-verbal reasoning skills, but also identified an attention deficit-hyperactivity disorder (ADHD). Psychopharmacological treatment had been of little or no benefit.

Sara's parents simply could not understand their daughter's inconsistent effort with regard to schoolwork and her refusal to accept the help of her teachers and tutors. Sara's teachers were also increasingly frustrated and angry. To be fair, it was also difficult for her therapist—and for me, as a consultant—to understand the tenacity of Sara's passive defiance. Sara seemed unaffected by her poor grades and by the efforts of her parents and teachers—whether through encouragement, cajoling, or punishment—to help her do her work. Many of her teachers thought that Sara was "manipulative." And Sara, like many children and adolescents, even when she was not overtly defensive, was unable to explain her lack of interest in her classes and her apparent indifference to the consequences of not doing her schoolwork. She would only say that doing her schoolwork did not seem "worth it."

Sara had also become defiant, disobeying family rules (for example, staying out beyond her curfew), with frequent outbursts of anger, especially toward her mother. Sara's parents felt anxious, angry, and ineffective, increasingly harsh in their reprimands and in their interrogations of Sara about her misbehavior, and more severe in the punishments they imposed. Sara felt that she was "different" and a "troublemaker" in her family.

Many of those attempting to help Sara—her teachers, her parents, and a previous psychological consultant—believed that Sara needed more consistent "consequences" for her failure to do her schoolwork. I disagreed. In my minority opinion, this apparently reasonable behavioral therapy would not help us understand or ameliorate Sara's demoralization ("it's not worth it") and was likely to harden her defiant attitudes and behavior. I recommended, instead, an empathic inquiry.

But this was not easy. Sara's therapist, Dr. P., described Sara as friendly, but emotionally distant, and Sara volunteered very little. She talked, with some animation, about her interests, especially reality television shows. But when Dr. P. asked about difficulties at home and, especially, at school, Sara responded with polite indifference. Somewhat later, Sara began to express resentment—of being "singled out" by teachers for her misbehavior—and also some disdain for her family's values. Why was it so important to be "smart" and to do well in school? Sara described to Dr. P. her experience of punishment by her parents. She complained not as much about being grounded, but about her parents' continuing anger at her after the punishment had ended, and her feeling that her parents could not really forgive her.

Sara's parents spoke with Dr. P. about their frustration with their daughter—her lack of interest in what was important to them and her unresponsiveness to their efforts to help. Mr. and Mrs. R. were perplexed—and themselves demoralized—by the ineffectiveness of their efforts. Dr. P. described the cycle of Sara's increasingly defiant behavior, her defiant response to criticism—whether expressed as apathy or anger—and the resulting intensification of their punishments. Dr. P. believed (and I agreed) that it was important to slow the sense of urgency Mr. and Mrs. R. felt about "fixing" Sara—and to find a way to open up more dialogue, to hear more of Sara's interests and concerns.

These discussions with Sara and her parents seemed to be helpful. Although Sara's schoolwork did not immediately improve, she became less defensive, more willing to discriminate between punishments that were fair and those that seemed extreme. The heatedness of family arguments began to dissipate, and Dr. P. was able to talk with Sara about her role in the cycle of poor performance and parental criticism.

Sara then showed some increased effort in her schoolwork. She expressed frustration, however, about seeing small gains for her effort. In this, Sara may have identified a core element of her difficulties—the problem of what sustains (and what erodes) interest and motivation. The causes of Sara's poor schoolwork were complex; despite her intelligence, Sara suffered intrinsic difficulties in focused attention and, over time, in response to criticism and disapproval, she had become disdainful and defiant. Fundamentally, however, Sara was demoralized. What enables any of us to put forth sustained effort—to work hard on difficult tasks—is the feeling that our effort will be "worth it," that our work will result in success—and recognition of success—that is commensurate with our effort. And, to Sara, schoolwork often seemed not worth it.

I cannot report that Sara's commitment to her schoolwork improved dramatically over the course of a year of treatment. However, Dr. P.'s thoughtful and patient efforts to promote empathic understanding in this family had been able to arrest (or at least to slow) a potentially malignant process of defiance and withdrawal—a significant therapeutic result. There were now many more moments when Sara felt appreciated in her family. She had become less defiant of family rules, less disdainful and withdrawn from other members of her family, and, in some measure, more open to help with schoolwork offered by her teachers. Dr. P. had hoped to do more—to continue to ameliorate Sara's defiant attitudes and, especially, to build on the opportunity offered by Sara's new openness to encourage the growth of her talents and interests, and to help her develop a more confident—and more realistic—sense of her intellectual abilities. As is often the case, the ultimate success of this therapy remains uncertain. Sara's family moved to California. Sara was enrolled in a private school that offered both academic support as well as strict oversight of homework assignments. Mr. and Mrs. R. were hopeful that this structure would be helpful to Sara, and Sara now seemed more willing to accept this help.

Notes

1. I suspect, from informal discussions with colleagues, that many therapists regard empathy simply as being "child friendly" or "nice" to patients, or worse, indulgent. A more substantive critique might argue—with some merit—that a clinical theory based on empathy fails to take into account the fundamentally interactive nature of the therapeutic process; and also fails to adequately describe the development of character, especially the role of conflict in character formation; and that a consistently empathic approach to treatment does not adequately challenge patients—including child patients—to change persistent maladaptive modes of thought and behavior.

   This is perhaps the most widely held view: that the therapist's empathy creates the conditions of acceptance and safety required in any therapeutic relationship and that expressions of empathy promote the child's willingness to participate in the real work of therapy, whether this involves, in psychodynamic models, the development of insight or the transformation of relational patterns, or, in cognitive-behavioral approaches, cognitive restructuring and problem-solving interventions. Only in the humanistic tradition (Wright, Everett, and Roisman, 1986) and in psychoanalytic self psychology (Ornstein, 1976) is empathy accorded a central therapeutic role, not only as a precondition to change, but as a primary *agent* of change.
2. This broad definition of empathy—as a mode of cognition that has evolved for the perception of affect and intention in others—is, I believe, a correct and useful one, and allows us to appreciate subtle expressions of empathy, both in parent-child relationships and in the therapeutic process. Some clinicians and researchers define empathy more narrowly, emphasizing the conscious cognitive component of empathy, and argue that empathy must include a conscious appraisal or understanding of another person's emotional state. On this basis, for example, Daniel Stern argued, in his now classic book, *The Interpersonal World of the Infant* (1985), that the important phenomenon of affect attunement, first described by Stern and which often occurs outside of awareness, is distinct from empathy. It is more helpful, however, especially when we consider the therapeutic process with children, to define empathy more broadly, and to regard any action that is responsive to the subjective experience of another person in a way that attempts to either mitigate distress or prolong positive affect, as an empathic communication. I therefore regard affect attunement as an early form of empathy.

3. Before we are too dismissive of the empathic capacity of other species, Bloom (2004) reminds us of experiments performed in the 1950s that demonstrated that monkeys (and even rats) will forgo eating if pressing a lever to obtain food also delivers a shock to a member of their own species. The monkeys will not starve themselves to death, however, and they had no inhibitions about shocking a member of another species (e.g., a rabbit) in order to receive food.
4. Halpern (2001) has presented a theory of clinical empathy in medical practice. In Halpern's analysis, clinical empathy begins with emotional resonance—the physician's immediate recognition and sharing of the patient's affective state. Emotional resonance, however, then requires "emotional reasoning" and imagination—an openness to memories and associations, what Halpern refers to as empathic "imagination work," that deepens the physician's appreciation of the nuances and unique meanings of the patient's emotional experience. Clinical empathy requires more than recognizing, for example, that a patient is angry; "empathy seeks to discern what, specifically, the patient feels angry about" (p. 79).
5. Demos adds that, in any given instance, although a caregiver may recognize a child's interest or distress, her ability to respond empathically is influenced by a variety of factors: her character and beliefs, the emotional support available to her, and the circumstances of the moment (for example, fatigue or competing concerns). Demos also adds an additional, important observation that continues to receive insufficient attention in discussions of empathy: an empathic parental response attempts both to reduce or end the infant's negative affective state and to facilitate or prolong the infant's positive affects of interest and enjoyment.
6. In a discussion of the therapeutic process in psychoanalysis, Blatt and Behrends (1987) describe this aspect of empathic communication as "giving voice to subtle personal experiences that the patient is struggling to articulate" (p. 287).
7. This effect has been studied experimentally in now classic "perturbation" research paradigms. Tronick (1989; 2006) and Stern (1985), by instructing parents to intentionally withhold or alter their normal emotionally expressive responses to their infants, have provided experimental demonstrations of the impact of this form of non-empathic behavior. In these experimental situations, infants experience evident behavioral and physiological stress. It is likely that chronic non-responsiveness leads to heightened physiological stress, increased behavioral withdrawal, and other, less readily observable and measurable inner psychological effects. Gottmann (1994), in his studies of marital communications, described an extreme form of this pathogenic process he called "stonewalling." These marital interactions are characterized by an absence of the non-verbal, "back-channel" feedback listeners normally provide to a speaker, non-verbal acknowledgments to the speaker that she has been heard. Gottmann's research demonstrates the severe consequences of these interactions for the marital relationship.
8. Schore (1994) has proposed that, in the very young child, these pathways are strengthened not only experientially, but also at a neurological level; that joyful interactions between parents and infants strengthen neural pathways between limbic and cortical brain structures.

8

The Problem of Resistance

In previous chapters, I have presented a general model of optimal and pathological development in childhood. In this model, the pathogenic process begins with some form of emotional injury—social rejection, academic failure, inability to elicit joyful responsiveness, harsh or persistent criticism. When normal reparative processes fail to mitigate these injuries, painful affects remain active in the mind of the child, leading to prolonged (or easily evoked) states of demoralization—withdrawal or defiant anger. I have compared this process to a malignancy: painful emotions, especially feelings of shame, resentment, and envy, become chronic aspects of the child's thoughts, fantasies, and behavior, intensify the child's always present inner conflicts, and increasingly shape the child's expectations of himself and others. And I have presented a corollary perspective on the therapeutic process, emphasizing the power of empathic understanding to arrest this malignant psychological development and set in motion a process of repair.

Clearly, however, this model does not solve all our clinical problems. Inevitably, we encounter the child's—and family's—resistance. It is a simple, but fundamental, clinical fact that children often do not want to talk to us about their bad feelings. Many parents consult us with the (not unreasonable) hope that this is our special skill—that, as child therapists, we will be able to do what they have been unable to do—to help their child "open up," tell them what is wrong, and talk to them. And parents often express concern about their child's general uncommunicativeness at home—the child's defensiveness and unwillingness to engage in dialogue, even to report mundane events of the day.

In a sense, of course, the parents are right: there is an art of child therapy and, as child therapists, we continually strive to perfect this art—to find, for each child, a unique blend of empathy and patience, playfulness and humor, that will help the child learn that talking about bad feelings *does* help—at least some of the time. Still, children tell even their most warm and accepting therapists—in response to our most tactful inquiries about their evident emotional distress or the events of past days and weeks, "I don't remember" or "I don't know." And even more strenuously, children do not want *us* to talk to *them*. Experienced child therapists, masters of their craft, routinely report that, "as usual, my words had little impact" (Yanof, 1996, p. 91).[1]

Resistance remains the nemesis of the child therapist. Children hide their bad feelings. And parents also, more or less stubbornly, continue to interact with their children in ways that we, as therapists, are likely to regard as destructive, hardening the child's demoralization and defiant attitudes, but that still feel profoundly "right" to them, an unquestioned tenet of their parenting "philosophy." Resistance is a limiting factor to the therapeutic power of the therapist's empathy; when resistant, the child does not let us in, or makes it difficult for us to convey our empathy, at least not in a straightforward way. When the child's or family's resistances are readily overcome, our task may be brief and relatively easy. More often, however, we need to find a way to "get through" (Taffel, 2001).[2] With both children and parents, an open acknowledgement of these problems and differences of opinion, from the beginning, is almost always a good place to start.

But why don't children want to talk with us about their bad feelings? Why do they so often tell us, when we clearly know otherwise, that, "Everything is fine?" Why do they put their fingers in their ears, or shout over us, ignore our questions, or say to us, "I'm not going to tell you" or "Shut up and play." Why do they so often refuse to listen to what we have to say? And what can we do about this? It may be helpful, in thinking about these problems, to keep in mind that children are not alone in their reluctance to acknowledge and talk about bad feelings. The child's expressions of resistance are perhaps less subtle than our own. But we all do this, to some degree—we hide our insecurity and self-doubt behind a multitude of avoidances and "reasons"—attitudes and behaviors we may stubbornly cling to, as do our children.

Overview

Before I suggest some answers to these clinical questions, I will again offer a brief review. Some experienced child therapists have warned that we may too readily consider a child "resistant"—that the child's resistances are often iatrogenic and labeling a child resistant may amount to "blaming the patient" (Lovinger, 1998). Others have argued that the concept of resistance is "an elaborate rationalization employed by therapists to explain their treatment failures" (Lazarus and Fay, 1982). There is, perhaps, some truth in these warnings. Child therapists may unwittingly exacerbate a child's resistance with too little playful interaction—too much talk and too many questions. In a more fundamental sense, however, the opinion expressed by Lazarus and Fay is certainly wrong. Some form of resistance—whether a resistance to talking openly or a resistance to attitude or behavior change—is encountered in every psychotherapy with children, including our most successful treatments. Resistance is more than an acknowledged practical problem for therapists of all schools (Leahy, 2001)—it is a manifestation of an instinctive and fundamental activity of the human mind, present, to some degree, at every moment of clinical interaction.[3] In everyday life, resistance is expressed in our reluctance to consider new ideas and in our opposition to anything that challenges our established sense of security. Resistance is the reason we so often fail to understand ourselves—and each other—and the reason that psychotherapy takes time.

I would propose the following definition: Resistance is the observable manifestation of the child's instinctive, self-protective actions *evoked by the anticipation of painful emotions.* Every emotional injury leads to some withdrawal and some strengthening of the child's protective shell. When these self-protective mechanisms are easily activated—when the child believes that talking about himself (and especially about his emotions) will be painful or dangerous—we will observe this in his behavior as defensiveness or vigilance.

Children's Resistances: Typical Forms

With this understanding in mind, let me return to our basic questions: Why are children so often reluctant to talk with us and what can we do about this? The child, of course, may have many reasons for not talking. For the sake of clarity, I will present, in outline form, the most frequently encountered resistances in child therapy. In most instances, a child's resistance is based on a combination of these reasons.

"Too Much Talk"

Children are afraid, not without some justification, that talking will make them "feel bad all over again." A child's bad feelings, of course, are not always present; for the moment, he may have established a tenuous, but good enough, emotional equilibrium—some relief from feeling "bad"—that he does not want threatened. If we would just leave him alone, he believes, his bad feelings will go away.

When we present this understanding to children—when we say, for example, "I think sometimes kids are afraid that if they talk about a problem, they're just going to feel bad... they don't want to feel bad all over again... they think that talking isn't going to help"—many children will acknowledge this fear. And, of course, we should admit, it is sometimes true, "When you talk about bad feelings, sometimes, for a minute, you *do* feel bad again." We can then add our opinion that, "It's still good to talk sometimes, because... then you can figure out a way to solve a problem... something that helps you feel better."

"There is Nothing Wrong with Me" ("I Don't Need to See a Therapist")

A child's fear that there is "something wrong" with him is perhaps his deepest resistance. These children may tell their parents, "I'm OK, I don't *need* to see a therapist." Often, the child *has* been told—explicitly and repeatedly—that there *is* something wrong with him (for example, when parents, in exasperation, have asked, "What is wrong with you?") or that he is "bad." At these moments, the child's resistance is motivated, at least in part, by the need to protect himself from a feeling of shame. For this reason, most children are more willing to talk about their *worries*, especially urgent anxieties or obsessive thoughts, because these feelings do not as directly threaten the child's self-esteem as, for example, a feeling of being rejected by peers.

These children cannot talk about painful feelings *because they are too painful*. They are afraid of what we might say to them, that we may confirm their unspoken anxiety—that there *is* something wrong with them—or that we might *blame* them (and they therefore vehemently blame others). When a child begins to sense in our questions, an implication—even a hint—that we think they have a *big* problem, not just *regular* problems that "a lot of kids have," he is likely to quickly become defensive, evasive, or refuse to talk.[4]

Protest and Argument

Children often refuse to talk to us as an act of protest or argument. Many children referred for therapy have been repeatedly criticized by their parents or teachers; and every criticism, or anticipation of criticism, evokes some defensiveness. By the time the child arrives at our office, criticism, argument, and unproductive discussion have become habitual; the child is now chronically defensive, engaged in ongoing inner argument. He anticipates more criticism, or he may be too angry to talk, or he may be angry at us. In these cases, the child's resistance is a form of protest—a private vow of silence.

Tommy, an 11-year-old boy with few friends, asked to know the name of the child whose session had preceded his. I felt uncomfortable with this possible violation of confidentiality, and in my somewhat clumsy explanation to Tommy of why I could not answer his question, I included the word "confidential." For several weeks following this brief discussion, Tommy refused to answer any questions *I asked*, replying, in a mocking tone, "That's confidential." This stubborn protest was symptomatic of Tommy's difficulties in his relationships with his teachers and peers. Although Tommy very much wanted to be liked and to have more friends, he pretended that he didn't care, and he would often respond to hurt feelings (or not getting what he wanted) with disdainful and supercilious verbal retaliation.

Talking Doesn't Help

Many children have developed a sense of futility about their family relationships—and a conviction that talking will not help. These children have often made some unsuccessful efforts to talk with their parents, to explain how they feel—especially, to convey feelings of unfairness. But the conversations have not gone well. The child's parents may have taken over the talking—and not spent enough time listening—and the child comes to believe that "talking" means being "talked to." Frequently, then, the child is right—talking has not helped.

There are still other motives for a child's resistance: He may be afraid of our disapproval (this is a variant of the child's fear that there is something wrong with him, or that we will think he is bad). Or he may need to protect a feeling of autonomy ("I want to do it myself"), again, a variant of resistance motivated by feelings of shame. Any statement by a therapist that challenges the child's established mode of coping with painful affects may also evoke resistance. Finally, we meet some children who don't seem to know how to talk about feelings at all. As a general rule, the tenacity of the child's resistance reflects the strength and depth of one or more of these factors—how much denial, for example, is necessary to protect the child from the shameful feeling that there is something wrong with him, or how much protest and argument have become habitual and pervasive in his emotional life.

What Can We Do?

With most children, we will have been able to mitigate the child's initial anxiety and resistance through our efforts at engagement: with our appropriately modulated, but still animated responsiveness to the child's interests and positive affects and our empathic recognition of his distress and grievance. These basic therapeutic attitudes—when we convey to the child, in words and actions, that we appreciate what is important to him—allow almost all children to engage with us in some, albeit sometimes brief, dialogue—about some problem in their life. And throughout the course of our work, general qualities of the child therapist—our patience, playfulness, and humor (and our willingness to talk about ourselves)—help most children begin to feel that talking about bad feelings is a normal and helpful thing to do, at least some of the time.

But we can do more. We can anticipate and speak with the child about all of his concerns. Every child who enters our office is anxious about what will take place. I find it helpful to openly acknowledge the child's anxiety and resistance from the very beginning. I may comment, for example, on first meeting a child, that he "must have been 'a little nervous' about coming to meet me; maybe, he didn't really *want* to come." Or I ask the child a first question, "So, what did you think about this idea of coming to talk to me today? Did you think it was a good idea? Or maybe, not such a good idea?" I let the child know that "a lot of times" children do not want to come to talk to me; especially, they don't like to talk about bad feelings. In this way, we "normalize" the child's resistance—we convey to children that their problems or bad feelings are problems *all* children, or *a lot* of children have. Somewhat later, I may comment that, "Sometimes kids don't want to talk because they think that talking won't help, or that talking will just make them feel bad again." And we should make sure to let the child know that we want to learn not only about their bad feelings—we want to know about their *good* feelings, too.[5]

When children are angry, we need to acknowledge the child's protest or defiant mood. Pine (1985) wisely recommends that we should limit our expectations of the child—of when and how much we would like the child to talk. I may tell a child that, "A lot of times, when kids feel bad about something, or when they are worried or angry, they say to themselves, 'I'm *not* going to talk about it.' But sometimes it helps to talk 'a little.'" Most often, once we have talked about a child's resistance on a given day, we have talked enough; it is enough to plant a seed and give the child some time.[6]

We need, especially, to be playful and to make use of humor. Once a child feels comfortable with us, if we ask too many questions, he may say, "Blah, blah, blah" as we begin to speak. In these instances, I may playfully pretend, "Oh, I know that language," and reply, "Blah *Blah,* Blah Blah." In a session that included the child's parents, a young boy began to speak in this way. His mother, somewhat embarrassed, admonished her son for his "disrespect." I, of course, was more accepting, and offered a simple translation, "I think that means that Jason is really annoyed at being asked so many questions about his feelings."

I sometimes like to pretend that I am a Jedi knight (or an evil Sith lord) who tries to use the Force to control a child's thoughts and actions; or that I recently bought a "mind reader" from a local store—a new invention that allows me to know what a child is thinking. Most children smile at this silliness and they are delighted that these devices never work—their powers can always defeat mine. Playfulness and humor are not magic—although our humor is often able to lighten the mood of the child's resistance, he will not immediately open up. But we have laid the groundwork for another time. We also offer children time-honored techniques for facilitating communication—children are often willing to draw, or write, or speak through puppets and action figures, instead of talk. But even then, when they write, they often write, "No talk."[7]

Is Anything Happening?

When we have acknowledged the child's initial anxiety and resistance and worked to create an affirming and responsive therapeutic setting, many children willingly, even eagerly, come to our offices to play—and briefly, to talk. After some initial discussions, however, although the child continues to play with enthusiasm, he is no longer willing to talk to us, often for extended periods of time. If we ask him why, he will complain that we "ask too many questions" (although we ask very few) or that we insist on "too much talk."

These are difficult moments for the child therapist. Those of us who continue to value and practice an open–ended therapeutic process (which still seems essential for most children who are chronically defiant or withdrawn, or have difficulty in their peer relationships) must honestly ask ourselves, is anything happening? Does the child need more time? Is this *therapeutic* play or merely "ritualized resistance?" (Chused, 2004) Or, is it both?

My experience suggests the following guidelines: If the child willingly comes to our office; if he plays with animation and enjoyment; if we understand the therapeutic possibilities inherent in interactive play—opportunities to promote emotion regulation and social development (Chapters 9 and 10); if, at the same time, we are working with his parents to foster more affirming parent-child relationships (Chapter 11); and if we continue to make ongoing assessments of the child's progress—improvements in the child's mood, behavior, and peer relationships—then we can be patient and trust the therapeutic possibilities of the play, as we try to create moments of dialogue and opportunities for the child to talk more openly with us about problems in his life.

Notes

1. It is largely in recognition of this fact that the technique of psychoanalytic play therapy was developed, considered by the first generation of child analysts as the equivalent of free association in the analysis of adults. We allow children expressive freedom in their play in the expectation that troubling feelings or fantasies will emerge in some form—in symbolism or metaphor, in the voices of characters in the narratives they create, in the roles they assign to us, or in more general aspects of the child's interaction with us. As Anna Freud recognized, however, even this is not sufficient. Children are reluctant patients and require our creative efforts to develop rapport, establish a working alliance, and help them talk about their bad feelings. Anna Freud (1946) succeeded, in some early cases, by making herself "interesting" to one child and "useful" to another.
2. Resistance is an acknowledged problem for child therapists of all schools, and our inability to successfully resolve a child's or family's resistance is the most common reason for therapeutic failure. Resistance on the part of children and parents is reflected in the high attrition rates that remain a significant problem for all child psychotherapy, including empirically supported treatment programs (Kazdin, 2005).
3. It may be helpful to recall, from an historical perspective, that the phenomenon of resistance was the first clinical fact Freud encountered as he abandoned the use of hypnosis and developed, in its place, the technique of free association. In an important sense, resistance—the patient's inability (or conscious unwillingness) to recall significant events or report his thoughts—is the origin and foundation of a psychoanalytic model of the mind. The inevitability of resistance in hysterical patients—that when asked to recall the events that led to the formation of her symptoms, the hysterical patient did not know and did not *want* to know—caused Freud to dissent from Breuer's "hypnoid" theory of hysteria and to formulate instead, the "cornerstone" concepts of psychoanalytic theory—censorship and defense (Freud, 1914).

Jonathan Lear (1992) has suggested that Freud's unique contribution to the philosophic tradition of self-examination and the injunction to "know thyself" was the concept of resistance—the idea that self-knowledge was not immediately available to introspection.

Michael Franz Basch (1982) has provided an excellent general statement of the contemporary psychodynamic understanding of resistance. Basch wrote, "For psychoanalysts and psychoanalytically-oriented psychotherapists, symptoms are not the indicators of what is wrong but are instead a demonstration of how the patient is trying to guard the vulnerable area of his emotional life and protect himself from further pain. Clearly, in most cases, these coping mechanisms will not readily be given up. Everyone of us in his character development comes to use various compensating and protective traits meant to fend off embarrassment, guilt, self-doubt, and other threats to his sense of integrity. . . . Whether they realize it or not, what our patients want from us is to be shown how to restore the balance that they had achieved without their having to make any fundamental changes in the way they see themselves and others" (p. 3).

4. There are times, of course, especially when we are concerned about the possibility of self-destructive behavior, when we need to ask questions that may evoke this resistance.
5. Recent experiments in social psychology have demonstrated what is perhaps intuitively obvious to all of us—that people are more willing to consider negative information if they are first presented positive information. When experimenters first provide some affirming experience (for example, experiences of success or recognition of acts of kindness) or induce positive mood in subjects, subjects are then more willing to consider negative information (Reed and Aspinwall, 1998). Following the induction of positive affect, for example, subjects are more willing to try new foods. These experiments and others also suggest a second conclusion, however, that is not intuitively obvious—that we are motivated not entirely by self-esteem enhancement, but rather by the need to maintain our self-esteem at a certain threshold; and that self-esteem may not be felt as closeness to the "desired self," but rather by distance from the "undesired self" (Ogilvie, 1987).
6. Pine offers other helpful recommendations, especially, that we allow children to anticipate disagreeable information. He explains, "with some children who hold their ears, screech, run out of the office, or break into panicky rage when something difficult is verbalized to them . . . I might say: 'Johnny, I want to tell you something you're not going to like hearing. I'll wait until after you finish that drawing and then I'll tell you' Or: 'Johnny, I have something important to say. Tell me when you're ready to hear it' (and then, after a while, since the child almost never tells one he's 'ready'): 'I'll wait five more minutes and then I'll tell you.' (I might add, 'You won't have to say anything, Johnny. I just want you to listen.') Or: 'Johnny, I have something a little scary to say, but it will take just a minute. After the checker game I'm going to tell you.' " (p. 155).

   A variant of Pine's approach is to set a time limit on how much we expect the child to talk. We can suggest to a child, for example, "Let's talk for five (or even two) minutes, then we can play." Even then, most children will attempt to negotiate our offer ("No, let's play first, then talk") and, if we agree (which I usually will), they will attempt to renegotiate when the time to talk has arrived. But we have made some progress—the child's resistance, although still stubborn, is now more playful and less strident.

7. For masterful case reports that illustrate a therapist's use of humor—especially, self-deprecatory humor—in softening a child's determined resistance, see King (1993) and Beren (1998). In a wonderful clinical essay titled, "Cookies for the Emperor," Robert King (1993) describes his therapeutic work with Guido, a 12-year-old boy in long-term hospital treatment. King reports that, "Guido spoke openly and directly about his problems" in his first session, but "he was rarely to do so again during the first year of treatment" and "large parts of hours would be taken up with seemingly sterile, repetitious play in which opposing warriors and armies endlessly annihilated one another." After many unsuccessful attempts to engage Guido in more direct dialogue, King asks one of the characters in Guido's fantasy play (Inspector H_2O) for help—to advise him on "a difficult case" of a boy who uses clever weapons to repel all of his inquiries. King reports, "The Inspector's advice proved very useful. In the guise of Inspector H_2O, Guido listened very seriously and said, 'Well, this is a very interesting case. It's clear he didn't get enough attention and affection growing up. He's having trouble getting started. He needs your help. He needs for you to kind of give him a little push to help him get started, show him you're friendly and he'll open up. I think he's just scared. He's scared his father will be cheated, or maybe that he will be cheated. I think you should just kind of let him know you like him and give him a chance. Make him comfortable, tell him to relax, and he'll come along'" (pp. 137–141).

   In a discussion of narcissistic pathology in children, Phyllis Beren (1998) describes her treatment of Jane, an eight-and-a-half-year-old girl who "did not make any effort at school and had difficulty completing her work. At home she had tantrums every day, usually about wanting her mother to buy her something special." Jane, however, "did not acknowledge having any problems...All she would grant is that her mother called her tantrums 'the fit of the day.' She herself had no idea why she had tantrums." Beren learns, in the course of her work with Jane, that "she was better able to tolerate my interventions if I used some humor or made a joke. Thus, I would preface my intervention with, 'Jane, you know that the only reason I am saying this is because it's my job. That's what therapists are supposed to do, to talk about the things nobody wants to talk about—but what can I do, it's my job; if I didn't do that, I would be out of a job.' This was often received with a big smile. She then allowed me to say, 'I know how you hate it when I suggest you might feel a certain way about something, because your mother is always telling you how she thinks you feel and that makes you so angry.' Jane could respond to this and say, 'You bet!'" (pp 152–155).

9

Child Psychotherapy as a Socializing Process I: Moral Development

For many children, especially those who present with impulsive or oppositional behavior, but often for withdrawn and anxious children as well, the child therapist has an inevitable, often explicit, socializing role. These children need to learn to control their aggression, to play by the rules, and to be able to make and keep friends. Perhaps the majority of children referred for psychotherapy require some improved socialization—improved behavioral control or improved peer relationships. Many of these children are sociable and engage easily with adults. In their homes, however, they are "noncompliant," unable to wait, and make frequent, insistent demands. Often, they do not play well with their peers. They may "overreact" with prolonged crying or anger when they are frustrated or disappointed, or when their feelings are hurt; or quit when things do not go their way; or disguise their anxiety and shame with bravado and braggadocio. They often prefer to play with younger children (or sometimes with older children from whom they more willingly accept an assigned role) and their circle of friends contracts.[1] Regardless of diagnosis, children who are unable to sustain friendships or who evoke frequent critical reactions from parents, teachers, and peers, are at high risk for increasingly severe emotional and behavioral problems in later childhood and adolescence.[2]

Again, the therapeutic process must intervene to arrest this malignant development. It is now generally recognized that individual play and talk therapy is not the treatment of choice for highly impulsive children and children with severe aggressive or disruptive behavior disorders. Programs of parent management training (Kazdin, 2005; Webster-Stratton and Reid, 2003) or parent therapy (Cavell, 2000) are an essential component of the treatment of children with conduct disorders.[3] Principles and techniques derived from these programs—especially the importance of positive parenting and frequent praise for incremental advances in the child's efforts at self-control and pro-social behavior—should be incorporated into a comprehensive approach to the treatment of children with problems of behavior regulation and social development (Chapters 11 and 12). Most school-age children referred for therapy, however, present complex problems of mood, behavior, and peer relationships (Cole and Zahn-Waxler, 1992). In my experience, these children benefit most from a treatment program that includes both individual psychotherapy and parent counseling.

In this chapter, I will present an integrative therapeutic perspective on the development of pro-social behavior in childhood. This perspective redefines problems of *behavior* as problems of *emotion regulation* (Cole and Zahn-Waxler, 1992; Gottman, Katz, and Hooven, 1997; Greene and Ablon, 2006; Malatesta-Magai, 1991). Every incremental advance in the child's ability to regulate her emotions—to feel sad, anxious, or angry without withdrawal, impulsive action, or unreasonable demands—will also result in improved social adjustment (Gottman, Katz, and Hooven, 1997). As a child becomes better able to tolerate disappointment and to bounce back from emotional distress, she will be more open to the socializing influence of parents and teachers—less "in the grip of" (Sullivan, 1953) painful affects and therefore more willing to listen to us. The child's desire or *want* is then less likely to become a *demand*, and her anxiety is less likely to be expressed as opposition or refusal. As she becomes less stuck in attitudes of blaming, argument, and denial, she will be more able to feel empathy and concern, to "take responsibility" for her actions, and to consider the needs of others. In contrast, social maturity does not develop in the presence of intense negative emotions. At these times, only a narrow focus—on the inner elaboration of painful affects or urgent efforts to get rid of bad feelings—is possible.

In addition to these critical processes of emotional maturity, my understanding of pro-social development in childhood also highlights the importance of the child's idealizations—her desire to *be like* admired adults—and the inherent socializing function of play (Panksepp, 1998). These elements of optimal socialization can be summarized in the following general thesis: Children most effectively learn essential social skills—cooperation, reciprocity, and the inhibition of aggressive behavior—in the context of pleasurable, interactive play with an admired adult who makes implicit and explicit behavioral demands. We learn an elementary lesson from our daily therapeutic interactions with children: Children seek playful engagement with adults who respond with enthusiasm to the child's interests and emerging skills, and who join in the game. It is in this context, I believe, that the child learns—deeply and committedly, not merely situautionally—(Kochanska, 2002) to accept the limitations imposed by adult authority. She must play by the rules so the game can go on.

Socialization: General Principles

Before I discuss how we can most effectively promote pro-social development in children with emotional and behavioral problems, it will be helpful to consider the process of socialization in a broader perspective. Socialization is an essential parental function. Children need to learn the skills and moral values that will enable them to take their place in adult society, "to love and to work," to become, in Louise Kaplan's (1986) apt phrase, "caregivers and lawgivers" to the next generation.

We are guided, fundamentally, in our efforts to socialize our children, by an image of the child's future—what kind of person we want our children to become and what children need to learn to successfully compete in the society in which they live. These images of the child's future shape the principles and philosophy of a family's socialization practices. We attempt to instill in our children qualities (virtues) and competencies that have become important to us—and that we believe will best ensure their future security and prepare them for future success.[4] These skills and moral qualities are regarded differently by different cultures, in different historical eras, and by different families, depending on the character and life circumstances of each parent.[5] World-wide, however, parents desire—and expect—their children to be sources of pride to their families.

In a frequently cited ethnographic study of working class mothers in South Baltimore, for example, Miller and Sperry (1987) report on the socialization practices of mothers in regard to the expression of anger and aggression in their daughters. These mothers, based on their own past and present life experience, had formed a core value and belief: their daughters needed to learn to defend themselves. The mothers' socialization practices were guided by this belief and intended to instill this survival skill. The mothers observed by Miller and Sperry frequently initiated teasing interactions with their daughters—interactions intended to give the child opportunities—and encourage her—to defend herself, "to practice fighting back" (p. 3). The authors conclude, "Qualities of strength, pride, and self-control figured importantly in [the mothers'] concepts of the mentally healthy child. The abilities to stand up for oneself and to 'take' pain and suffering without betraying hurt feelings were highly valued" (p. 15). "What emerges is an ideology that emphasizes the need to "toughen" the young child through practices such as teasing" (p. 10).

These values were also conveyed in the language used by the mothers and in the stories they told their children or when the children were present. When these mothers talked to their children about incidents of threats or actual physical abuse by men, they did not mention fear or vulnerability, but focused instead on the need to retaliate when justified and to not be a "sissy" or "spoiled." Miller and Sperry also note, of course, that toughness was not the only quality valued by these mothers—affection, nurturance, and sympathy were also valued and taught, "each in its own place" (p. 16).[6]

Parental socialization practices are also determined by a second set of beliefs—beliefs about *how* important life lessons and qualities of character are best learned, what Miller and Sperry call a "folk theory" of child rearing. This research has important implications for our therapeutic work with families. We need to understand, and take into account, the guiding values and beliefs that parents hold—beliefs about *what* is important for their child to learn and about *how* children learn these necessary life lessons.

Among the forms of behavior that are especially subject to parental socializing efforts in childhood are the regulation of aggression, the recognition of status and authority, the expression of emotions, and gender differences (i.e., how boys and girls, men and women, should behave). Moral socialization involves the development of inhibitory behavioral controls—especially the control of aggressive and sexual behavior—and a recognition of the rights of others, embodied in rules or law ("Thou shalt not..."). Behaviorally, the young child learns what is permitted and not permitted (for example, no hitting or swearing); what is expected and praised; and what is punished or disapproved of. Children are also socialized to become members of a social group. Successful socialization promotes a sense of belonging and an acceptance of the obligations to others that are part of being a member of a social group.[7]

These guiding principles are filtered through the character of the parents—especially, how they have come to cope with the demands of being a parent. The actions of parents toward their children will therefore be determined both by an implicit parenting philosophy and by how well parents are able to manage their own anxiety and anger. Parents who feel frustrated, preoccupied, insecure, or unappreciated will be less likely to respond with enthusiastic interest or playful responsiveness when their children seek them out for fun; or with empathy and patience when their children are anxious or upset; and they are especially likely to be *reactive*, rather than *proactive* in their interactions with their children. If we are able to appreciate both the *concerns* of parents—what is important to them—and the demands of their own lives, we are more likely to help them find a balance of playfulness and encouragement as well as prohibitions—to be both an authority *and* a friend—that promotes the successful socialization of their children.

Socialization: Theory and Research

In normal development, how does optimal socialization occur? Behaviorist principles have been the dominant theoretical and clinical paradigm for understanding the socializing process. An implicit behaviorist perspective remains widely practiced as a therapeutic model, especially in the advice we offer parents. A behaviorist approach to moral socialization, however, although useful if understood in the larger emotional context of parent-child relations, has been challenged by recent clinical and developmental research.

Behaviorist theories of socialization rest on the fundamental principle of reward and punishment. Children are rewarded, with praise and approval, or more tangible rewards, for desired behavior; and punished, with disapproval or removal of rewards, for undesired behavior. The child learns what is permitted and not permitted—and to inhibit undesired behavior—because of the *consequences* of his actions. Based on this general model, it is commonly assumed that the child's acceptance of adult authority depends on the consistency with which that authority is exercised; that is, the consistency of the parents' demands and their enforcement of sanctions or "consequences."

This basic behavioral principle is widely, perhaps universally, accepted, and, to some extent, it is universally true. Fear of punishment—later internalized as conscience—is important in the development of every child. And this is the advice most commonly offered to parents—by therapists and in the public media: to be consistent in the rules they establish and the consequences they impose. This model includes a corollary assumption: that children will behave badly, that they will challenge or defy adult authority, when it "works"—when they are able to avoid facing the consequences of their actions, when they have learned that they can "get away with it." In this account, the child—and all of us—makes some, perhaps implicit, calculation of the immediate and long-term consequences of her actions and then behaves accordingly.

There is, of course, some self-evident truth in this theory. Optimal socialization, however, includes more than the child's acceptance of adult authority and compliance with adult demands. Most parents hope to instill in their children feelings of empathy and concern for others (Winnicott, 1963; Eisenberg, 2000), of appreciation and gratitude, and a desire for giving, not simply taking or getting. It is now increasingly recognized that successful socialization involves much more than consistent rewards and punishments, except perhaps in the broadest sense.

Parental Pride and the Development of Ideals

The psychoanalytic theory of socialization adds to the behaviorist model the concepts of identification and the development of an ego ideal. In the classical psychoanalytic theory presented by Karl Abraham (1921/1927), acceptance of adult authority begins when the child exchanges primary physical pleasures for the (socialized) compensation of finding pleasure in adult approval. The child substitutes a moral satisfaction (i.e., being a good boy or a good girl) for an instinctual satisfaction (e.g., harming a younger sibling). This model highlights not only the child's fear of punishment and disapproval but also her wish *to be like* an admired parent or parent surrogate, what Chassequet-Smirgel (1985) has called the "project" of identification. In the psychoanalytic theory of development, optimal socialization also involves the child's successful transition from the pleasure principle to the reality principle, from the age of illusion and imagination to the age of reality.

The young child's idealization of her parents (and of older children) is among the most readily observable facts of childhood. Young children look up to their parents with a feeling of awe that is difficult to recapture in adult life (except perhaps in a religious person's experience of God). The young child believes that her parents know everything and can do anything. Kohut (1966) proposed that these early idealizations are gradually transformed, through a process of "optimal disillusionment," into the adult's capacity for commitment to guiding ideals. Again, I believe, Kohut has identified a profound developmental truth: that, despite the inevitable disillusionments of adolescence, parents should remain, in some way, to some degree, idealizable—admired or respected—and that the preservation of ideals in some form is essential to emotional health. Kohut suggests that, in the absence of ideals, specific forms of psychopathology develop, for example, cynicism, nihilism, or an urgent search for ideals.

In this theory of socialization, children seek recognition and affirmation from admired adults who then become a guiding influence. All children want their parents to be proud of them—as parents want to be proud of their children—and the internalization of parental pride is a fundamental socializing influence. Expressions of pride from admired adults evoke in the child a unique and essential good feeling. This feeling is then "internalized" as an expectation, promotes acceptance of adult demands, and becomes a sustaining influence in moments of disappointment, discouragement, and temptation. In contrast, parental criticism or derogation breeds resentment and defiance, and undermines the development of guiding ideals. In my clinical experience, the child's acceptance of rules and learning of reciprocity, although certainly influenced by fear of punishment, is at least equally dependent on the internalization of parental pride.

This dimension of pro-social development is largely neglected, even among psychoanalytic child therapists, and especially in our advice to parents. Many parents fail to appreciate the critical importance of the child's idealizations—as a sustaining influence in the child's emotional health and in the successful socialization of their children. We need to help parents more frequently express pride in their children and appreciation of their child's efforts toward pro-social behavior.

Emotion and Moral Development

Early research on the socialization of children focused on the consequences of different parental disciplinary styles (e.g., democratic versus authoritarian) on children's social and moral development. (For an historical review, see Maccoby, 2007). Although disciplinary practices remain important (especially parents' ability to minimize harshly punitive or coercive discipline), there is now considerable research support for the role of emotions—parental responsiveness to the child's emotions, parental expressions of positive emotions, emotional conversation and dialogue, and emotion "coaching"—in the moral and social development of children. Several decades of socialization research supports the conclusion that moral development proceeds not as much from fear of consequences, but from learning of reciprocity.

In a study reported over 20 years ago by Parpal and Maccoby (1985), for example, mothers were briefly trained (in one 15- to 20-minute training session) to engage with their 3- to 4-year-old children in responsive play for 10 to 15 minutes each night. The child was allowed to choose any activity and to control the nature and rules of the interaction. Mothers were instructed not to praise the child, "but rather, to participate positively in the child's play... to describe and imitate her child's behavior, to comply with her child's directives... [and] to let the child know that she enjoyed playing" (p. 1329). Just one week later, the children of these mothers were observed, in an experimental session, to more willingly comply with their parents' requests than children of mothers in other experimental conditions who had not received this training. Parpal and Maccoby also report that this brief training in responsive play seemed to have had its greatest effect on "difficult" or hyperactive children.[8]

In a study of the mother-child relationship as a source of support or stress, Dumas and LaFreniere (1993) observed that what distinguished the interactions of socially competent preschool children and their mothers (in contrast to children rated by their teachers as anxious, aggressive, or average in their social skills) was higher levels of "positiveness"—laughter, helping, approving, and expressions of positive affect—words of endearment and affectionate gestures.[9]

Kochanska (2002) has recently proposed a theory of moral socialization focusing on the development and internalization of a "moral self" in childhood. Kochanska and her colleagues have distinguished two distinct forms of compliant behavior in young children. "Committed compliance" is characterized by the child's expressions of "satisfaction, pride, and positive emotion while complying; the child's compliance has a voluntary, autonomous quality, is accompanied by positive affect and pride, and seems to come 'from inside.'" In contrast, "situational compliance," although essentially cooperative, "is contingent on sustained maternal control" (p. 339). Based on observations of young children in both naturalistic and experimental situations, Kochanska proposed a model of internalization for boys (the findings did not apply to young girls), consistent with contemporary psychoanalytic theory, in which "boys incorporated their experiences during the instances of eager, enthusiastic, committed compliance into their future views of themselves as highly moral individuals, or 'good' children. Such moral selves then became a guiding regulatory system for moral conduct" (p. 347). In contrast, situational compliance remained "situational" and did not lead to the construction of a "moral self."

Emotion Coaching

The research of John Gottman and his colleagues (Hooven, Gottman, and Katz, 1995; Gottman, Katz, and Hooven, 1997) on emotional communication in families has special relevance to the child therapist and provides compelling empirical support for the role of both empathy and emotion regulation in child development. This research may take on even greater importance in light of recent evidence (summarized by Sapolsky, 1996) on the damaging effect of prolonged stress on brain functioning. Gottman and his colleagues describe a critical developmental pathway—a pathway that begins with parental acceptance and "coaching" of children's emotions, leading to improved physiological and emotion regulation, and then to improved peer relationships, especially conflict-resolution skills.

Based on both parent interviews and direct observations of parent-child interactions, Gotttman and his colleagues identified differences, among normally functioning families, in parental philosophy regarding the experience and expression of emotion, especially expressions of anger and sadness. The parents' attitudes and behaviors with regard to emotions—their thoughts and feelings *about* feelings—constitute what Gottman, Katz, and Hooven call a family's "meta-emotion" structure. Gottman described a style of parental communication and interaction he labeled "Emotion Coaching." Emotion coaching parents valued emotions. They more often acknowledged and talked with their children about feelings and encouraged the expression of anger and sadness by their children. In contrast, non–emotion coaching parents, although they were not "bad parents," were more often dismissive or derogatory in regard to their children's expressions of emotion.[10]

Gottman, Katz, and Hooven present detailed results on the relationship of family meta-emotion structure and children's adjustment. An emotion coaching meta-emotion family structure was associated, at ages 5 and 8, with multiple positive child outcomes, including better academic achievement, more successful peer relationships, and lower levels of stress hormones. In contrast, parental "derogation"—expressions of criticism, mockery, and contempt (especially by fathers)—was strongly associated with negative outcomes for children. These results were summarized in a developmental pathways model of adaptive functioning in childhood that highlights the child's increasing capacity for emotion regulation. Gottman, Katz, and Hooven suggest that social (and academic) competence in childhood depends on the development of a set of *emotional* skills; especially important is the child's ability to regulate her emotions sufficiently to be able to listen to what another child is saying, and then to engage in joint problem-solving. An emotion coaching style of parental communication leads, most directly, to improved physiological regulation; reduced physiological arousal allows improved attentional skills and more flexible responses in peer interactions—"the ability to resolve conflict, to find a sustained common ground play activity, and to empathize with a peer in distress" (p. 101)—and therefore more successful peer relationships. In this model, emotion regulation—especially the ability to inhibit expressions of negative affect (for example, aggression, whining, or oppositional behavior)—is the essential social skill on which the development of other social skills depends. Gottman, Katz, and Hooven suggest that, "being teased in middle childhood is the ultimate proving ground for the child's ability to inhibit negative affect" (p. 101).[11]

The Inherent Socializing Function of Play

From the beginning, play has been regarded as the primary expressive medium of child psychotherapy. The first generation of child analysts valued the child's fantasy play for its potential symbolic content, allowing the expression of inhibited affects, memories, and desires—desires the child senses as a threat to her security or conscience. More recently, child therapists of all schools have recognized additional therapeutic benefits of interactive play. In a seminal essay, Slade (1994) illustrated the therapeutic value of "simply playing" with young children. Slade, and many others, observed that interactive play with troubled children, accompanied by minimal interpretation, often leads to significant emotional and behavioral improvement—expanded narrative development, increased affect tolerance, and increased compliance at home and at school.[12] Frankel (1998) has described therapeutic play with children as an opportunity for "recognition" and "renegotiation of self-other relationships through action."

All of these processes are observable in therapeutic play with children: expression of inhibited feelings and wishes, elaboration and "renegotiation" of interpersonal narratives, and the development of increased tolerance for frustration and disappointment. But there is more. Socialization is always happening in the course of interactive play. Every moment of interactive play with an admired adult offers opportunities for pro-social development. The child is learning, experientially, the limits of verbal and physical aggression and the need to make accommodations to others, that she cannot, for example, push too hard and must wait her turn.

Panksepp (1998) argues that play is an instinctive, "signature mammalian behavior," subserved by basic neural structures shared by all mammals. Mammals housed in isolation are hungry for play, and "humans are a uniquely playful species" (p. 287). Panskepp suggests that different forms of human play, including joking and verbal banter, reflect "variations on a primal theme, complex elaborations of a basic play instinct that generates a diversity of behaviors" (p. 286). The hallmark expression of play circuitry in humans is *laughter*, an emotional expression that may have evolved as a social signal of victory, group solidarity, or safety.

Panksepp presents evidence to support the hypothesis that, among the many functions and benefits of play, in most mammalian species, play

> . . . may allow young animals to be effectively assimilated into the structures of their society. This requires knowing who they can bully and who can bully them. One must also identify individuals with whom one can develop cooperative relationships and those whom one should avoid. Play probably allows animals to develop effective courting skills and parenting skills, as well as increasing their effectiveness in various aspects of aggression, including knowledge of how to accept defeat gracefully. (p. 280)

In rats, play has been demonstrated to increase gene expression and to activate areas of the cortex involved in pro-social development. Panksepp also presents preliminary evidence that (again, in rats) abundant opportunities for play may reduce, to some extent, the impulsivity that results from frontal lobe lesions (Panksepp, 2001) and he offers the intriguing hypothesis that, in children, an impoverishment of play and playfulness may intensify the child's materialism (and, I would add, demandingness); that is, the child asks for "things" as a substitute for playful interactions.

Consider, in summary, the following psychological benefits of interactive play:

(1) Interactive play provides opportunities for shared positive affects of interest and excitement.

(2) Interactive play provides opportunities for modulated, socialized expressions of defiance and aggression, for example, teasing. Dunn and Brown (1991), in their observations of patterns of communication between parents and young children, note the early emergence of joking and teasing in both parent-child and sibling relationships. Teasing by children was clearly evident in these interactions at age 24 months. "The essence of teasing is provoking an emotional reaction in another, and the delight of children in their success is all too evident, even in their second year" (p. 102). Dunn and Brown suggest that "a plausible case can surely be made that such interchanges are important to learning the acceptable limits of insult, criticism, or expression of dislike in a significant emotional relationship" (p. 101). My clinical experience supports this hypothesis. Teasing emerges frequently in therapeutic play with children. And, as Dunn and Brown report, the child's pleasure in teasing us—hiding, laughing at our errors, pointing out our ineptness, even playful cheating—is "all too evident."

(3) Moments of anxiety, frustration, and disappointment inevitably occur in the course of interactive play. This is true of both fantasy play and, especially, of structured games—a toy is broken or missing; a tower accidentally falls; the child's spin or roll of the dice does not land her on the space that she wants. These moments provide a therapeutic opening: as we talk with the child about her frustration and disappointment, and offer some solace and consolation, the child develops an increment of tolerance for anxiety and frustration, and a measure of emotional and behavioral flexibility, and of problem-solving.

(4) Interactive play provides opportunities for the child to learn accommodation and reciprocity. In play, accommodation to the other person is always necessary and learned experientially.

(5) Adult play with children involves an inherent socializing influence—these interactions provide almost continual opportunities for the child to learn rules and limits. Every playful interaction—with a parent or therapist—necessarily involves some subtle limit or prohibition. If we are playing catch, neither player can throw too hard; in play fighting, the child cannot hurt her

opponent. In these interactions, the child comes to understand and accept—deeply and for the right reasons—that rules are necessary—for safety and for living with others. These socializing influences do not occur in *solitary* play. In our offices, in our homes, and in every group activity, this is how children learn to accept rules and limits—experientially, in the context of intrinsically rewarding play.

It is important to note that these interventions are not essentially didactic. To the dismay of many well-intentioned parents, most children do not learn socialized behavior from repeated "talks" or lectures. Adult intervention is effective because the rule must be observed *in order to continue the play*.[13]

Jason: Teasing

Jason is a 6-year-old boy, referred for therapy because of episodic aggressive behavior, both at home at school. At times, with minimal apparent provocation, Jason would become explosively angry—punch other children, pick up a chair and threaten to throw it at another student, or threaten to jump out of a school window. Several months would pass without incident, and during this time, Jason was generally happy and playful. Still, although infrequent, these incidents were alarming and dangerous. (I noted a seizure-like quality to Jason's explosiveness; neurological examinations, however, were negative.) Jason's therapy involved many elements: discussions of traumatic events he had witnessed; exploration (together with his parents) of the context and precipitants of his aggression; active encouragement of different ways of *being* angry—what Jason could do when he began to feel angry; and involvement of school personnel in both a therapeutic and an emergency plan to promote regulated, appropriate expression of anger and to protect Jason's safety and the safety of other children.

Jason, however, also loved to play, and he often felt that we had talked too much. At these times, he would ignore my most benign comments and questions, or respond in a sing-song, "Blah, blah..." When we played, Jason would begin playing according to the established rules of the game; if I gained an advantage, however, he would cheat—blatantly, without any effort at concealment. If we were playing chess, Jason would make an illegal move and capture my Queen, and then a Rook. Soon, he would have every piece and I would have none. Jason did not play this way in every game and he did not show the full cheating syndrome (Chapter 10). At times, he was able to "accept defeat gracefully" and I learned from his parents that Jason never cheated when he played in real life. In our sessions, however, Jason could not help himself—cheating was just too much fun.

When I commented on Jason's obvious cheating ("Hey, I think you just took my guy"), Jason would teasingly answer, "No, I didn't, that must have been another kid." He would then laugh—heartily—as he soon "won" the game. And I could not help laughing, too. I then made a suggestion at the beginning of each new game ("Hey, Jason, what do you think, should we play without cheating this time?") and Jason would often agree, "Yeah, I think we should." He promised, with mock seriousness, not to cheat; and then, when I gained an advantage, he would laugh and cheat again.

But this was no longer serious or urgent cheating. It was teasing—roughhousing with chess pieces—a playful form of aggression and a kind of playful interaction that this young boy had rarely, if ever, experienced with his volatile, emotionally remote, and, at times, verbally abusive father.

Notes

1. Children who require improved socialization are heterogeneous, with one common characteristic: they have difficulty regulating their emotional reactions. One group of children very frequently referred for treatment are impulsive; these children have also been described as "strong-willed" (Forehand and Long, 1996) or "explosive" (Greene, 1998; Greene and Ablon, 2006) and may be diagnosed with ADHD, oppositional defiant disorder, or childhood bipolar disorder. Other children present some degree of impairment in social cognition and social relatedness, often diagnosed with a non-verbal learning disability or Asperger's syndrome.
2. It seems necessary to raise an essential question: Why are we having so much trouble socializing our children? Is the prevalence of these childhood problems the result of more frequent biological insult and risk? Or do we now place greater—and perhaps unreasonable—demands on our children for focused attention and early academic achievement, causing unnecessary frustration and discouragement? The effect of children's vastly increased time spent in passive electronic stimulation (Singer and Singer, 2005) and decreased opportunities for interactive play is clearly cause for concern. Many have noted the diffusion and breakdown of support formerly available to children from extended family members and from religious and community affiliations. Or are there other, unidentified causes?
3. Several successful and promising treatment programs have been developed for children with severe or early-onset oppositional defiant disorder and conduct disorder (Kazdin, 2005; Webster-Stratton and Reid, 2003) and aggressive behavior (Lochman et al. 2006; Greenberg, 2006; Cavell, 2000). There are, of course, significant differences among the various parent management training programs that have been presented and tested. Recent approaches to parent training focus less on "consequences"—teaching parents how to impose effective sanctions for a child's non-compliance and misbehavior—and highlight, instead, the importance of frequent praise. See Cavell (2000) and Greene and Ablon (2006) for discussions of empirical limitations as well as empirical support for these treatments.
4. Erikson's (1950) anthropological studies, although now generally regarded as incorrect in his hypotheses regarding the impact of specific child-rearing practices on the formation of adult character, illustrate this general principle. In the Sioux tribes studied by Erikson, for example, where the role and "identity" of being a successful hunter was essential to survival, parents

attempt to instill in their children the skills (e.g., endurance and endurance of pain) and virtues (e.g., cooperation, leadership) required for the success of the child and the survival of the community, embodied in the society's ideals.

This process is perhaps most evident in the indoctrination practices of totalitarian, ideological societies. In Nazi Germany, children and adolescents were socialized (indoctrinated) to inculcate the militarist and racial supremacist ideology of the Third Reich. In Communist Cuba, children of school age are taught the values of Che Guevara's "Socialist Man"—an ideal citizen who values commitment to society over individual achievement.

In the history of psychology, the most famous (or infamous) example of this principle is John Watson's (1928) advice to parents. Watson warned parents that they should not kiss or hug their children. This "coddling," Watson believed, would create dependency and "invalidism"—a whining, unhappy child and, later, an adult who would be unable to tolerate discomfort, persist in constructive activities, or overcome difficulties on her own.

Or consider a more recent example. Jamie Foxx, in his controversial 2005 Academy Award acceptance speech, spoke approvingly of his grandmother's efforts (that included corporal punishment) to help him become "a Southern gentleman." "She was my first acting teacher... she told me, 'act like a man.'"

5. LeVine (1974) proposed three child rearing goals shared by parents in all cultures—what parents want *for* (not *from*) their children: (1) physical survival; (2) that their children become economically self-sufficient; and (3) the acquisition of cultural values. In LeVine's analysis, child rearing customs "represent adaptations to environmental pressures experienced by earlier generations of parents seeking to realize the universal goals of parenthood... means by which parents have responded adaptively to their experience of environmental hazards threatening the health and future welfare of their children" (p. 239). LeVine suggests that cultural variation in the priority of these goals is largely determined by economic conditions. He notes, for example, that obedience (as opposed to independence or self-reliance) is more highly valued as a child-rearing goal among Western working-class families and in non-Western agricultural societies than among more affluent Western families and in hunting and gathering economies. "Parents [in working-class and agricultural societies] see obedience as the means by which their children will be able to establish themselves economically in young adulthood when the basis must be laid for the economic security of their nascent families. Thus parents who emphasize obedience are anticipating the occupational demands their children will face" (p. 237). When parents believe that their children's economic future is more secure, obedience loses some importance as a child-rearing goal and "parents can evolve child-rearing philosophies and fashions that are less tightly coupled to the hazards of economic failure" (p. 237). LeVine notes that parents may not be consciously aware of the relationship between subsistence conditions and child-rearing values, which have become embodied in cultural customs (and, I would add, in Western societies, parental character.)
6. Parental socialization of the child—parents' efforts to mold the child and instill virtues—may begin (unconsciously) even earlier, before the child is born, as early as choosing a child's name. Parents choose names that convey,

for example, the importance of respect for traditions, or alternately, the cultivation of individuality (D. Brooks, 2007).

Active parental socialization efforts intensify dramatically in the second year of life, as the child becomes able to separate and explore. These early socialization efforts have the purpose of keeping the child safe from harm. Schore (1998) reports that whereas "at 10 months, 90% of maternal behavior consists of affection, play, and caregiving… the mother of a 13–17 month old toddler expresses a prohibition on the average of every nine minutes" (p. 64).

This basic parental function, most readily apparent in early childhood, continues beyond childhood. Parents continue to teach their children to identify the dangers they will encounter—initially, threats to their physical survival and, later, threats to their psychological well-being and to the survival of their social group. Parents make some effort to alert their children and keep them away, as adolescents and young adults, from the dangers of the external world, and to keep them close—at first physically close, then close in a broader sense, for example, through adherence to traditions. These instinctive socializing efforts by parents are a frequent, perhaps universal, source of conflict between parents and children, especially in adolescence, as the child's desire for exploration clashes with her parents' concern for safety and security.

7. Processes of socialization also occur, not only in families, but within all social groups (including professions) and the basic principles are the same: group members are taught—and required to demonstrate—behaviors and values essential to the survival of the institution and its members.
8. Parpal and Maccoby plausibly interpret these results to support a "reciprocity" theory of behavioral compliance versus a social deprivation or social reinforcement theory. Their concise conclusion is worth noting and has significant implications for the advice that, as child therapists, we offer parents: "Although we do not question the likelihood that Skinnerian processes can bring about changes in children's immediate compliance under some conditions, our results point to an entirely different set of processes. The 'responsive parenting' manipulation employed here did not involve reinforcing children for compliance, or giving them negative feedback for noncompliance" (p. 1332). Parpal and Macoby also review previous research that supports a reciprocity theory of compliance—research that demonstrates that even very young children are more likely to comply with their parents' requests when parents have complied with the *child's* requests.
9. The authors report that "mothers of socially competent preschool children, when observed in interactions with their children, were more positive (in behavior and affect) than all other mothers" (p. 1740). Mothers in this study, however, also seemed to reinforce their children's pro-social behavior. "Whenever competent children behaved positively, their mothers were likely to immediately reciprocate positively" (p. 1750). Dumas and LaFreniere also report that, unlike all other children, competent children tended to respond to (rather than ignore) their mother's expressions of disapproval.
10. Gottman, Katz, and Hooven also observed parents teaching their child to play a video (Atari) game. Emotion coaching parents were more engaged (versus disengaged) with the child, issued positively worded instructions ("Do" versus "Don't do" statements), were more responsive to the child's questions, and less

intrusive in their behavior (for example, grabbing the joystick). These parents also expressed more affection, enthusiasm, and humor; non-emotion coaching parents expressed more criticism, anger, and derisive humor.

11. Thompson, Laible, and Ontai (2003) report an important series of studies that provide additional support for the role of emotion regulation in moral development and extend Gottman's findings. In these studies, the best predictors of children's early moral development were not references by parents to rules and consequences, but, instead, a parent-child relationship characterized by shared positive affect and an "elaborative" conversational style, in which mothers made frequent references to other people's feelings. Thompson, Laible, and Ontai distinguish "elaborative" conversation from "pragmatic" conversation. Elaborative conversation is similar to Gottman's description of emotion coaching. In contrast, pragmatic conversation is characterized by "short, directive conversations centered on specific events or questions that invite a simple 'yes' or 'no' response" (p. 149).
12. See also Bromfield (2007), Cohen and Solnit (1993), and Singer (1993).
13. Panksepp (2007) reminds us that Plato regarded this process as an essential component of the socialization of children. In the course of children's play, Plato observed, a bully emerges. At these moments, adults intervene to protect the safety of all children and this adult intervention socializes the potential bully.

10

Child Psychotherapy as a Socializing Process II: Winning and Losing

This chapter continues my discussion of psychotherapy as a socializing process, taking up one of the most common problems encountered in child therapy—winning and losing at games. To facilitate engagement with child patients and to lessen the burden of excessive or potentially threatening inquiry, child therapists have traditionally offered the child an opportunity to play structured games. Many children readily accept this offer. If the child is a boy, he is likely to eagerly anticipate these contests—and he will arrange to win, at least most of the time.

We learn a first lesson from playing games with young children: how important it is for them to win. For most children seen in psychotherapy, these games *matter*. The child does not *want* to win; he *needs* to win. Winning, by whatever means, evokes in the young child a feeling of pride; losing evokes a feeling of failure and shame. It would be difficult to overestimate the importance of these emotions in the psychological development of the child, perhaps especially young boys.[1] These children take great pleasure in their victory—and our defeat. To insure their victory, they make up their own rules, changing them for their purposes and to their advantage during the course of the game. As the child begins to sense that winning is possible, especially in the setting of safety we have established, he is unable—with more or less playfulness and knowing smiles—to restrain the impulse to cheat or to change the rules, to make his victory certain. Often, they are not content with winning, but also engage in some expression of gleeful triumph—boasting, bragging, and taunting. This behavior, described in a classic essay, published almost 40 years ago, by John Meeks (1970) can still be observed with unchanged regularity.[2]

Why do boys referred for psychotherapy need to play with us in this way? We can perhaps easily understand the child's urgent need to win. But why do they insist, not only on victory, but on gleeful triumph? Perhaps the answer to this question is simply that this is what young boys are like: the child's jubilant behavior is an instinctive expression of pride, derived from displays of social dominance readily observable in non-human primates, an undisguised expression of a basic competitive need of human beings (both men and women)—to be better, in some way, than someone else.[3] For boys, the feeling of *winning*—the need to feel a sense of physical or intellectual dominance, to display their strength and skill, to feel strong in relation to other boys and men—seems essential to their self-esteem. Young children need to believe that they can—and will—do great things.[4]

If we are honest, we will have to admit that the child's need for competitive triumph is never completely outgrown. Competitive success is a fundamental principle, continues throughout life, and seems to confer some evolutionary advantage. As adults, our expressions of triumph and superiority, because of our fear of public disapproval, become more muted or disguised. And our ability to cope with failure and defeat, both in childhood and as adults, is in many respects, a measure of our emotional maturity.[5] But we are still allowed, and still need, to celebrate our victories.[6]

Losing, to all children, feels painful. To many children referred for psychotherapy, losing feels catastrophic, and they respond with behavior reminiscent of the "catastrophic reaction" classically observed in brain-injured patients. Often, it does not seem to matter whether the game is a game of skill or a game of chance. If the child loses, he may throw game pieces, insist on a "do over," or refuse to play. In these cases, we suspect that the child urgently and insistently needs to win in order to compensate for chronic feelings of demoralization or defeat, especially academic failure or social exclusion. (In his essay, Meeks also noted the frequent occurrence of the cheating syndrome in children with learning disabilities.) But, to be fair, we all get caught up in the game.

Many children who play in this way, both boys and girls, are temperamentally impulsive and strong-willed. It has therefore been more difficult for them to learn to modulate their expressions of frustration and disappointment, and they often respond to other disappointments (for example, losing a cap or being denied a treat or a souvenir) with the same catastrophic feeling as losing a game. Some younger children have not yet emerged from the age of illusion, the age when children are not yet expected to fully understand the idea of rules.

"Mommy, I Cheated, I Won"

Matthew is a 4-year-old boy whose hyperactive and noncompliant behavior ("not listening") had reduced his thoughtful and caring parents to tears—and to their wit's end. In our first meeting, Matthew chose to play Candyland. Like so many children with whom I have played this first game of childhood, Matthew picked the cards he wanted from the deck, discarded those he didn't, and quickly landed on the winning square. He then ran excitedly into the waiting room to brag about his success, "Mommy, I cheated, I won." (In subsequent sessions, Matthew and I built robots, using Legos. Matthew took great delight in our "battles," as his robots routinely smashed mine into smaller and smaller bits.)

Such statements from a 4-year-old are charming, and most parents can tell similar tales of their young child's blithe indifference to rules—and of the resentment and envy evoked in older siblings who have entered a new developmental stage—the age of reality. (When the parent of a 3-year-old appropriately expresses effusive praise for the child's early attempts at drawing, a 6-year-old sibling is likely to respond, "That's not beautiful, that's a scribble.") But the persistence of magical, illusory play, beyond the age of illusion, into the school years, reflects a developmental failure of socialization that is likely to have significant consequences for the child's peer relationships and emotional adjustment. Successful peer relationships depend on learning to play by the rules.

Losing and Demoralization

Most children who cheat and brag are also demoralized—they are not "winners" in the "playground politics" (Greenspan, 1993) of childhood. In real life, these children fall apart when they lose; they may choose to play with younger children who they can more easily dominate or control, or they may avoid competition altogether. From a behavioral point of view, it may be said that these children have not learned mature or appropriate social behavior and this description is, of course, true. More fundamentally, however, these children—in their peer and family relationships—feel, in some way, defeated. Winning—and boasting—offers temporary relief from chronic feelings of shame—failure, defeat, and envy.

Tom, an anxious 10-year-old boy, in one of our first sessions, asked to play chess. Tom won our first game. But, in the second game, I won. Tom became tearful. Despite my best efforts to offer support and understanding—about his good play and my many years of experience—Tom remained, for a long time, inconsolable. Later, I spoke with Tom's father about this experience. Mr. G. told me that he had often observed the same reaction, especially when he played tennis with his son. Tom, he explained, was not yet good enough to beat him. When he loses, Tom cries or becomes sullen and leaves the court, and Mr. G. is highly critical of Tom for his "immature" behavior. The father, of course, is right—his son is not yet good enough to beat him (and the child knows this) and Tom's behavior is immature. Still, I was taken aback and privately cringed at the unmitigated toughness of Mr. G.'s attitude. Tom felt defeated and demoralized. (In school, Tom was also demoralized by the impact of learning problems.) Mr. G. seemed not to have recognized this and, as a result, Tom had become increasingly dismissive and defiant in his attitudes toward his father.

I would object less, or perhaps not at all, if Mr. G. had tempered the reality of his superiority with some effort to mitigate Tom's defeat and offered explicit appreciation of every advance of the child toward increased competence and skill. Tom might then anticipate the day when he would win fairly, as did a somewhat older child, who told his father, with warmth and admiration, "I can't wait until I can beat you at tennis." In the end, this may be what is most important—a parent's encouraging, generative attitude toward competitive play with the child.

A Therapeutic Opportunity

But is there any *therapeutic* purpose served in playing these games? (Or, how can we make this game play therapeutic?)[7] In my opinion, the therapeutic goal of playing games with children is to promote an essential aspect of successful socialization: to enable the child to play (and to work)—without quitting and without cheating. This critical aspect of emotional maturity depends on the child's ability to tolerate moments of anxiety, frustration, and disappointment—moments that are inevitably present in any constructive activity. In child development, the problem of cheating, and even gloating, needs to be redefined—not as a moral problem but as a problem of affect tolerance. The child cheats because, in that moment, he cannot bear the feeling of losing; he urgently needs to win, and we can help him most effectively if we understand the urgency of this feeling.

Meeks offered several wise (although, at the time, controversial) recommendations for the therapeutic management of the cheating syndrome. He advised that we allow the full expression of the child's cheating; that we express praise ("barely short of flattery") for every increment of real skill; and that we acknowledge our own past shortcomings and failures. Eventually, Meeks believed, the therapist would be able to help the child understand the ultimate futility of cheating—that a reliance on cheating interferes with the achievement of real skill and a legitimate feeling of pride.

I would offer some additional recommendations. When playing games with children in psychotherapy, we should approach the play with an empathic understanding of the importance to the child of winning and losing and an appreciation of the game's socializing function. We need to remind ourselves that, often, the child is not yet playing a game—his play lies somewhere in-between fantasy play and a true game. With this understanding as a guide, we can then develop a good-natured and incremental approach to promoting the child's social development—his acceptance of rules and the rights of others.

We first observe how the child engages in the game. How seriously does the child play and how insistently does he attempt to control all aspects of the game, for example, which piece he chooses or who goes first? How does he respond to minor frustrations and disappointments that occur during the play? How urgently does he need to win? In the course of playing a game, as in anything we do, there are inevitable moments of excitement, anxiety, frustration, and disappointment. When we play with children, if we play with enough enthusiasm—and express some of our own excitement and disappointment—the child will also, in some way, acknowledge these feelings. These brief moments—of anxiety and, at times, defeat—present a therapeutic opportunity: we are able to observe, in vivo, how the child attempts to cope with frustration and disappointment, and talk with him about it.

Therapeutic game play with children, of whatever age, therefore consists of an ongoing conversation about feelings—as much as the child will allow. In the course of these games, I talk with children about how much kids *really want* to win, about how *good* it feels to win, and how *bad* it feels to lose; about how much fun it is to "slaughter" me; and about the feelings of anxiety, frustration, and disappointment that occur, if only briefly, as the game proceeds. And that we all have these feelings. I may say to the child, "I think a lot of times kids feel really bad when they lose... maybe that's why kids cheat sometimes... I think everybody feels bad when they lose." Depending on the age of the child, I may add, "Sometimes I feel a little bad, too, when I lose. Because it feels really good to win. But then I say to myself, 'I think I might win the next time.'" And we offer consolations—especially consolations that offer the promise of future success (as, for example, when we point out to a child who has tried, but failed, to catch a ball, that he "almost" caught it) and, as Meeks advised, we offer explicit praise for each increment of effort and skill.

In this way, an empathic parent or therapist promotes an essential aspect of ego development and successful socialization—a future orientation. Even if defeat feels terrible now, the child will not always lose.

Expanding the Conversation

As we talk about the child's feelings—how it feels to win and to lose—we are often able to expand the conversation. We may learn about the unfavorable comparisons the child makes between himself and others—the friends he envies because they "always" win or the "geniuses" in his family. He may eventually tell us, "I have to win when I play here... because at school (or in my family) I always lose." Most children seem to derive some benefit from talking about the disappointments and frustrations endured by their heroes - baseball players, for example, who sometimes strike out, that even the best players suffer disappointment and defeat. (It has often been noted that, in baseball, the best hitters fail twice as often as they succeed.) Our goal in these discussions is to promote small increments in the child's ability to tolerate disappointment—to feel disappointment as disappointment, not as catastrophe, and to learn that he will not *always* win or *always* lose.

With children who continue to cheat for extended periods of time, we will need, at some point, to introduce reality considerations into the play and challenge the child to play by the rules. I find it helpful to begin tentatively and playfully, to suggest to the child that we cannot always play "their way." Many children, however, with more or less insistence, resist this idea; their intransigence reflects a developmental failure in the socializing process. Or a child may accept—in theory—the principle of "no cheating"; but during the game, if he begins to lose, he will be unable to resist the impulse to cheat. Our response should then be good-natured. I smile when the child cheats, and say, "Hey, you cheated." His cheating provides us, again, with a therapeutic opportunity—to talk about how it feels to win and to lose.

As we continue to encourage more reciprocal, rule-governed play, we offer the child some negotiation and compromise, for example, "Let's play one game your way, then one time the regular way" or "You can go first this time, then it's my turn to go first." (In my office, in the first game we play each day, the child always goes first, because he is my guest.) For children who are especially inflexible, we may need to begin with even simpler, less consequential, challenges and negotiations, for example, "This time, I think I want the green pieces."

When playing games of skill, where it is apparent to the child that we have superior knowledge and experience, we do not play "our hardest." We can play with a handicap, or not play competitively at all, or point out to the child that he has made a bad move and let him take it back and try again. It is a sign of therapeutic progress when the child tells us, "Play your hardest"—evidence of increasing maturity, acceptance of reality, and the desire to "really" win (although, in the heat of the battle, he may still regress and, again, resort to cheating.)

In my experience, it is generally unnecessary to go farther than this. We have already accomplished some increment in the child's acceptance of disappointment, his ability to bounce back from defeat and, with this, some improvement in his ability to successfully play with others. We may learn from the child's parents that, although he continues to cheat when playing with us, he no longer cheats in real life. Or, the next game, he will cheat again, but more playfully—perhaps with a smile—and if we ask him why he continues to cheat, he will tell us, "Because it's fun."

Variations on a Theme

Although the cheating syndrome is remarkably typical of young boys in therapy, there are still many variations on the theme. Lawrence, an impulsive and often oppositional 7-year-old boy, is playing Chutes and Ladders. When his spin does not land him on the square he wants, Lawrence spins again. I comment, "I think sometimes kids feel really disappointed when they have to go down that chute, because they really want to win." Lawrence makes no reference to what I have said; he continues to cheat and, eventually, to "win." My comment, however, seems to have had some impact. In our next game, when I land on the same square and must go down the chute, Lawrence tells me, "It's OK, *you* can cheat." This is a clever compromise and a significant developmental advance: an implicit recognition of the need for fair play and concern for the feelings of the other player. Lawrence wants to make amends for his cheating (but still reserve the right to cheat). When working with some withdrawn children (for example, John, Chapter 6), we may need to allow the child to win, for long periods of time, and even welcome the emergence of cheating, as an indication of increased spontaneity and freedom of expression—a freeing up of inhibition.

At times, however, more explicit socializing influence is required. If, despite our empathic and educative efforts, the child's cheating remains triumphant or hurtful—if his taunting continues to go "over the line"—we may need to establish a prohibition and enforce a consequence. At these times, I will tell the child, "If you make the other person (i.e., myself) feel bad, we will have to stop playing for a few minutes" (just as we do when other basic rules are broken). Tommy was an 11-year-old boy whose taunting of me was especially hurtful and relentless. (Tommy's refusal to answer questions was discussed in Chapter 8.) Tommy loved history, so we wrote a "Constitution" together—and added Amendments—concerning the rules of our games.

I am often asked, by parents and students, an unavoidable question: Should we let the child win? Over time, I have arrived at a simple answer: "Yes, but not every time." What is more important, I believe, is this: If, as a parent or therapist, we play often enough and with enough enthusiasm—with at least some attention to the child's pleasure in winning and some effort to soften his disappointment when he loses—the question of letting the child win becomes less urgent. With each advance in the child's ability to tolerate disappointment, as his self-esteem is no longer shattered by losing, he becomes more open to our socializing influence, less insistent on playing *his* way, and, eventually, to "accept defeat gracefully."

There is one additional—and, perhaps, most important—aspect of this dimension of socialization and emotional development. Although it is difficult to be certain, I have often found that, among the factors that contribute to the problem of cheating—and other problems of moral socialization—is some failure in the child's relationship with his father. The father may have been absent, or angry and critical, or himself unable to gracefully accept defeat. This aspect of the child's emotional life is difficult to observe—children will only occasionally tell us about it. But a child's learning to play by the rules may largely depend on the knowledge that those he admires—and whose approval remains important to him—also play by the rules. In the absence of this guiding influence, the child's adherence to rules is likely to remain tenuous and "situational."

What Can Parents Do?

The problem of cheating is more difficult for parents, who do not have the luxury of a therapeutic setting and must insist, more firmly than we do, on playing by the rules. Some parents, in frustration, have given up playing with their children. However, if we are able to help parents begin to understand the problem of cheating as we do: based on the instinctive importance of *winning* and the child's need to compensate for feelings of demoralization—to be a "winner" and not a "loser"—and requiring an incremental approach to the development of reality constraints, we can provide some guidance. I recommend that parents play frequently and enthusiastically with their child, and allow the child to play "his way"—sometimes, but not every time. In these playful, competitive interactions, in innumerable small experiences of victory, followed by defeat, followed by victory, losing becomes tolerable.

Are there risks in this incremental approach to socialization and the adherence to rules? Are we indulging the child, promoting a false and maladaptive view of life, encouraging a sense of entitlement that might reinforce a child's demanding attitudes and behavior ("No, I want it *my* way! It has to be *my* way!"). I believe this risk is minimal. I will often smile or laugh as a child blatantly cheats, but there are always rules and always limits. The child cannot hit me, or throw game pieces, and he must help me put away our games.

Peter: "How Can This Be?"

Peter is a 6-year-old boy, referred for treatment because of frequent, prolonged temper tantrums, often triggered by common, expectable frustrations and disappointments. In his kindergarten class, Peter might cry, at times for almost an hour, if he was not chosen to be first for an assignment; at other times, he might become angry and throw something; or lie on the floor, pulling his hair; or he would sit at his desk, crying quietly.

Peter had been a very "difficult" infant and toddler, emotionally intense, with a high energy level and short attention span. Psychological testing highlighted significant difficulties, characteristic of children with attention deficit-hyperactivity disorder (ADHD), on tests of focused attention, working memory, and impulsivity; mild deficits were also noted on tests of phonological processing. Medicine was prescribed, with some success, particularly in reducing Peter's impulsivity and general disinhibition.

Peter's parents seemed somewhat less sensitive or sophisticated than most in many of the common ways parents help young children tolerate or "bear" the expectable frustrations and disappointments of early childhood. Peter's father, skeptical of soft-minded psychology in general and play therapy in particular, accepted my evaluation and recommendations reluctantly. Peter, he believed, needed more discipline than his wife was able to provide. His tough-minded approach was, from my point of view, short on expressions of pride; but he was also capable of playfulness and encouragement, and he was never, to my knowledge, harshly critical, certainly not abusive or demeaning, toward his son. There was humor and fun, as well as strictness, in this family.

Because of the pervasive nature of Peter's emotional crises, I understood Peter's difficulties as a disorder of affect tolerance, requiring a kind of developmental help. Peter experienced ordinary disappointments not as *disappointments,* but as calamities or *injustices*. Peter's teachers, with some urgency, wanted to know what to do. I encouraged them to anticipate and make note of moments of disappointment, to label these feelings and talk with Peter about them, and to actively support, with praise, small increments in Peter's ability to "handle" his emotions. (I should have, at the same time, encouraged more playful interactions and positive affect sharing in Peter's family; however, I did not yet fully appreciate the therapeutic benefit of these interactions.)

Peter's difficulties quickly became apparent in therapy sessions. As the end of each session approached, Peter began to protest, "No, just one more game; It's not fair; I didn't have enough time"; often, he refused to leave the office. He might grab his cheeks in frustration, saying, "Oh no! How can this be?"

I tried to help Peter anticipate these moments, and we talked about them, as much as Peter would allow ("All right, c'mon, I know, you're wasting my time"). I told Peter that I understood his frustration and disappointment and offered consolations ("... next time"); but, at the end of the hour, Peter's protest emerged almost without diminution ("I don't want to stop; I used to get more time; I'm so mad I want to rip my shirt and pants... life is so difficult"). I also told Peter about times when I had felt sad and very angry and how I had tried to make myself feel better; this session ended calmly, with Peter more accepting of his disappointment.

Peter played with intensity; he loved to play and he needed to win. The crisis of the previous hour did not seem to dampen his enthusiasm or eagerness for our next opportunity to play. Over time, these end-of-session crises diminished; Peter's difficulties continued, however, with equal intensity, but in a new form. Peter liked to play a variety of board games, particularly military games. He approached these "games" with a predetermined plan to defeat me and he would cheat, blatantly, so that his plan would succeed. If his spin, or roll of the dice, did not land on the space he wanted, Peter would spin again. Occasionally, at times by chance, at other times as part of a planned attempt to test the possibility of helping Peter move toward a more reciprocal form of play, I would gain a small advantage or, still at a disadvantage, capture a piece he had not intended me to capture. Peter became furious ("*so* angry"); he would implore me to allow him a "do over"; if I did not immediately agree, Peter would throw his pieces, threaten to break the game, or pull his hair. Again we talked, often over Peter's vehement protest ("Stop talking, let's just play") and we negotiated. (For example, I suggested to Peter that if he began to feel upset, he could tell me and *then* peek at my pieces). I did not insist on playing by the rules. But these are difficult choices for the child therapist; when (and how) do we exert socializing pressure and challenge the patient (gently, of course, and often with humor) toward greater acceptance of reality constraints and recognition of others?

I realized, somewhat belatedly, that Peter was not yet playing a "game"; his intention was something closer to fantasy play, with game pieces in lieu of action figures. I explained this to Peter and he seemed to feel understood (this meant, of course, that we would continue to play "his way"). This form of play, however, had by now continued well past the age of normal illusion or omnipotence and posed a serious obstacle to Peter's developing satisfying relationships with peers.

I asked, on one occasion, how things were going at school; Peter answered, indicating his understanding of the therapy process, "Hey, you're here to help me be a good person, not to talk." I accepted Peter's supervision and generally limited my comments to the affects that emerged in the course of our play. I noted, and verbalized, Peter's increasing excitement in anticipation of victory, as well as brief moments of anxiety and frustration (more typically, of course, there was an absence of anxiety, and instead, a grandiose sense of invincibility). I hoped, in this way, to broaden the range (particularly the mid-range) and complexity of Peter's affective experience (see Pine, 1979, on the "expansion of the affect array") beyond the extremes of gleeful triumph and abject defeat.

Peter's rage in sessions became less frequent, tempered by increased self-awareness and even some humor. Peter's parents reported dramatic improvement in "real life." Peter's tantrums in school had stopped. He joined a baseball team and, when he struck out, he did not cry. Despite this considerable improvement, I remained concerned. Peter still did not have many friends or a best friend. Although we had accomplished a lot, I cautioned against ending Peter's therapy. Peter also did not want to stop. So we continued, at reduced frequency, until Peter's family relocated several months later.

Notes

1. And in human relations generally. In benign or malignant forms, the emotions of pride and shame are critical determinants of human attitudes and behavior. Throughout life, we want to be winners, to identify with winners, and avoid "losers." An essential aspect of the appeal of many tyrants, despite their ruthlessness, is their ability to undo feelings of humiliation and provide a renewed sense of national or ethnic pride. (Recall that Hitler promised to restore pride to a defeated German nation.) Or consider a less consequential example: many fans of the San Francisco Giants—but few baseball fans elsewhere—are willing to forgive the cheating of Barry Bonds, because his records give them pride.
2. Citing an earlier article by Peller, Meeks contrasts the "oedipal" play of the preschool child, characterized by a prevailing mood "of triumph [and] of a naïve invincibility" with the seriousness and rule-governed play typical of school-age children, who, in normal development, understand the game as an opportunity to test and improve their skill against a worthy opponent.

3. I have asked many children, while engaged in these playful "competitions," to "help me understand something about kids: Why do kids need to win all the time and why do they sometimes need to cheat?" The answers to my questions, unfortunately, have not been especially revealing. The child most often replies, in the same spirit as the play, "Because I want to" or "Because it's fun."

   Bloom (2004) presents an analysis of laughter that may help us understand the child's triumphant laughing and taunting ("Ha ha, I win, you lose"). He reminds us that, "gangs of monkeys make laughter-like sounds when they attack a common enemy. And chimpanzees, like humans, make laughing sounds when acting in mock aggression" (p. 184). Bloom argues that cruelty is intrinsic to humor and that humor involves this essential element: "someone is knocked off a pedestal, brought down a peg."
4. Erik Erikson, in *Childhood and Society* (1950) tells of his conversation with a young Sioux boy who boasted that "he could catch a wild rabbit on foot and with his bare hands." Erikson gently laughed (*with*, he thought, not *at* the boy) and "I was made to feel that I had made a social blunder. Such daydreams are not 'play.' They are the preparations for skills which, in turn, assure the development of... identity" (pp. 142–143). Harter (1988), in her interviews with pre-school children, reports a similar finding. "In the very young child, one typically encounters a fantasied self possessing a staggering array of abilities, virtues, and talents. Our preschool subjects, for example, gave fantastic accounts of their running and climbing capabilities, their knowledge of words and numbers, as well as their virtuosity in winning friends and influencing others (Harter and Pike, 1984). For example, fully 50% of them describe themselves as the fastest runner in their peer group" (p. 122).
5. From the point of view child development, especially the emotional health of the child, the philosophy of Vince Lombardi (*"Winning isn't everything, it's the only thing")* is profoundly wrong. There is much more that makes competition an important socializing experience: learning to be a member of a team, learning our commitment to others, and, especially, learning to play by the rules. Children need to learn that rules—whether in games or in families, in schools, or in other institutions—are not essentially arbitrary or capricious. Although rules may seem arbitrary to children, they are there for a reason. Families and communities need to demonstrate these reasons to their children. (Of course, it is also true that rules may be unfair—especially when they are exclusionary, promote bias, and enforce gender and social class distinctions—and then need to be challenged and changed.)
6. Not all boys, of course, brag or show off in this way, and this may reflect successful socialization and emotional maturity. I have worked with some children (and adults), however, who were unable to celebrate their victories (or other achievements). In these cases, the inability to celebrate was an inhibition or a symptom of depression, and the child's need for competitive success found some alternate form of expression, especially as moral and intellectual superiority, or in the child's fantasies and dreams.
7. There is some controversy about the usefulness of structured games as a therapeutic activity. Some child therapists—and perhaps many parents as well—warn that playing games with children can too readily become a convenient resistance for both the child and his therapist, and there is some merit in this critique. I agree, however, with Bellinson (2002) that we should

play these games with children. When playing games becomes an ongoing resistance, these children are likely to be equally resistant to any effort we make to help them talk about behavioral problems or painful affects. Moreover, games are important to most children of school age. Important affects and self-evaluative processes accompany the play, and the way the child plays (especially how he wins and loses) opens up, for therapeutic intervention, essential aspects of his emotional development and sense of self. So, for better or worse, I have spent a considerable amount of time playing games with children. And it seems to be my lot as a child therapist to be roundly defeated by many of my young patients—in imaginative play by very young children, in structured games by somewhat older children, and in intellectual competition by still older children and adolescents. We learn, of course, to accept these defeats "gracefully" and to compensate for our humiliation at the hands of the child with some therapeutic and theoretical yield.

Part III

Parent Guidance

11

Parent Guidance I: Promoting Emotional Health and Resilience

Goals of Parent Guidance

In previous chapters, I have presented a malignancy model of child psychopathology and a resilience model of children's emotional health. This perspective on emotional development has important implications for parent guidance—how we can best help parents help their children. With some important exceptions, advice to parents offered by psychologists, in both the popular and professional literature, remains largely behavioral, focused on methods of discipline—"shaping" pro-social behavior and teaching parents how to impose effective sanctions when children misbehave—with the goal of achieving improved "compliance" with parental demands.[1]

Although compliant behavior (especially, "committed" compliance, Chapter 9) is an important concern of most families, a resilience model of emotional development suggests a broader set of goals for parent guidance. From this perspective, the guiding principle of therapeutic work with parents is the repair and strengthening of parent-child relationships. We enlist parents' active participation in an effort to (1) identify and ameliorate vicious cycles of negative parent-child interactions; (2) restore affirming responsiveness between parents and their children; and (3) promote parental behaviors that strengthen the child's positive expectations—expectations that sustain initiative and problem-solving, and reduce the child's avoidance and withdrawal. Behavioral compliance is a subsidiary goal, and best achieved when we are able to help parents reestablish a family atmosphere of affirmation and support.

Effective parent guidance requires that we establish—and then sustain—an alliance with parents in working toward these therapeutic goals. In this effort, it is helpful to keep in mind that being a parent is among the most joyful and rewarding, but also the most demanding, of life tasks. And raising a child with a difficult temperament, a child who is impulsive or hyperactive, strong-willed or given to negative moods, is especially demanding, "a litmus test for parental foibles" (Cole and Zahn-Waxler, 1992, p. 187). In his review of the role of positive emotions in child development, Robert Emde (1991) reminds us of the joyfulness that almost all parents experience at the birth of an infant. For too many families, this joy quickly fades, as parents struggle with the physical and emotional stress of child rearing. Raising children in contemporary American society, despite our affluence, is, arguably, emotionally more difficult than at other times and other places. Modern parents, because of the diffusion or breakdown of extended family networks and other social supports, may have less help available to them—help that has traditionally been available to parents—as they attempt to cope with the demands and uncertainties all parents face in caring for their children. Both parents and children now have fewer places to turn when they are in need of solace and emotional support.

Parent guidance begins in the initial consultation. In these first conversations, we initiate a collaborative process of inquiry and exploration. Our inquiry will lead to a diagnosis (Chapter 5), but goes beyond diagnosis, as we develop working hypotheses about the causes of the child's problematic moods and behavior. Often, we will learn of traumatic or injurious events in the child's life—experiences of loss or illness, separation or divorce—and it is essential to understand the impact of these events in the life of a child and family. It is equally important, however, to identify present, ongoing pathogenic processes—daily experiences in the lives of children (for example, marital and parent-child conflict, bullying or exclusion, frustration in learning) that we may be able to more quickly ameliorate. Our emerging understanding will, in almost every instance, include an appreciation of the child's temperament—especially problems of sustained attention and impulsivity, specific learning difficulties, or anxiety sensitivity—and how these qualities of temperament, in interaction with parental responses, have set in motion vicious cycles of defiance and withdrawal. And we need to understand the demands faced by parents, individually and as a family, and communicate an appreciation of the parents' values and concerns. Our empathy must extend not only to the child, but (to the extent possible) to her parents as well.[2]

As parents describe recurrent problematic moments in the life of their family, it is important to learn, in as much detail as possible, the sequence of interactions that occurs and the opinions of all family members—the context of these moments, triggering events, the child's behavior, and parental reactions. But we should not forget to inquire beyond these problematic interactions—we also need to learn about the child's interests and abilities and what parents and children enjoy together.[3]

A Therapeutic Plan for Families

Based on this emerging understanding, I present to parents, early in the treatment process, a therapeutic "plan"—a set of recommendations, tailored to the concerns and problems of a particular family—to arrest pathogenic family processes, strengthen family relationships, and promote the child's emotional resilience. These recommendations typically begin with an effort at increased empathic understanding of the child—a new or deeper appreciation of the anxiety, frustration, or discouragement that underlies the child's problematic behavior. But we must also offer immediate practical help—active strategies that address parents' most urgent concerns and begin to ameliorate recurrent problematic situations. When parents feel that they have a plan—that they know what to do, for example, when a child is disrespectful, ignores their requests, or refuses to go to school—they will be less anxious and less *reactive* in their behavior toward their child. Any recommendation we are able to offer that increases a parent's confidence in his ability to handle his child's emotional crises (including his ability to enforce reasonable rules and limits) may therefore have other beneficial effects as well.

In developing a therapeutic plan for families, child therapists should consider these essential steps:

(1) We begin with a respectful appreciation of parents' anxieties and concerns—their goals for their children (which we are likely to share) and their efforts to promote their child's success in life. Although, in most cases, we will offer parents a new understanding of their child (for example, that "lazy" and "controlling" are never adequate explanations of a child's behavior) and recommend new ways of responding to their child's difficult behaviors, we also need to acknowledge parents' strengths as parents, especially their genuine concern for their children, and what they are doing right as parents, not just what we believe they are doing wrong. And parents also have grievances—legitimate reasons for their anxiety and anger. Parents need to know that their child's therapist understands their frustration with the child's tantrums or defiance.[4]

Many parents welcome our new understanding and readily accept our recommendations; others remain skeptical. To some parents, our focus on the child's emotions (and only secondarily on the child's behavior), our willingness to compromise (in an effort to teach compromise) and to engage the child in active problem-solving (in order to teach problem-solving), may seem to be the wrong lessons, too much "giving in" to the child's demands, at odds, in some important respect, with their parenting philosophy (or, in other cases, simply impractical). A parent's skepticism must be discussed as openly and fully as possible, in an effort to arrive at some mutual understanding. Parents may then find a way to incorporate our ideas in a way that works for them. It is not always possible to resolve these differences. However, if we gloss over a parent's disagreement, our success will be severely limited—or parents may abruptly terminate the child's therapy.

(2) We offer parents a new understanding of the sources of the child's distress—especially, greater appreciation of the child's anxiety, frustration, or discouragement. And we educate parents about how demoralization and defiance have come to be expressed in the child's moods and behavior.

(3) We attempt to identify—and then ameliorate—ongoing patterns of family interactions that perpetuate painful emotions in the mind of the

child, especially vicious cycles of criticism and defiance. We help parents understand the *importance of reparative moments* in the life of the child—and the need for parents to initiate this repair.

(4) We work with parents to find opportunities for responsiveness to their child's interests and to create more moments of positive affect sharing in their daily interactions with their children.

(5) We teach and encourage proactive problem-solving (Greene and Ablon, 2006) and support for the child's pro-social behavior.

(6) We help parents find ways to combat the child's demoralization and foster—in small increments—improved self-confidence and self-esteem. In moments when their child is disappointed, discouraged, or angry, we help parents restore for the child a positive sense of herself and her future, to recognize and express appreciation of the child's strengths, and to develop what Wachtel (2001), in an important contribution, has called "a language of becoming."

(7) Finally, we help parents establish reasonable rules and enforceable sanctions for violations of these rules—rules that protect the child's safety and respect the rights of others.

Positive Affect Sharing

A parent's increased responsiveness to a child's interests and positive emotions is a first step in the strengthening and repair of parent-child relationships. Taking into account the character and life circumstances of each parent, we encourage parents to create moments of positive affect sharing, especially in the form of animated play—play that is responsive to the child's interests and her emerging skills.

Young children are almost always eager for this kind of "attention" from their parents. (Our task is more difficult with adolescents who have become defiant and withdrawn, and who may no longer *seem* to care.) I therefore ask parents, in every initial consultation, "What does your child like to do?" and "Is there some way that you can more frequently share this interest with her?" I encourage parents to more frequently and more actively share in their child's interests—to find a form of responsive engagement that works for them—on a daily basis, beyond being present at the child's performances and athletic events, and to set aside some time, every day, to *play* with their child. Especially for young children, it is important for parents to play with enthusiasm and genuine enjoyment—whether they join their child in building with blocks or Legos, in fantasy play with dolls or action figures, in zooming cars or airplanes, in organizing the child's collections, in rough and tumble play, or exploring a children's Web site.

We learn, again, an elementary lesson from our experience as child therapists (and as parents): Children eagerly anticipate sharing their interests. When parents are able to engage with their children in this way—with more frequent and more enthusiastic play (and playfulness) and to respond with *interest* to their child's *interests*—the child will look forward to playing with her parent and essential psychological benefits regularly follow: an expansion of the child's interests and imagination, a strengthening of the child's expectation of affirming responsiveness, and greater willingness to make accommodations to others. The immediate behavioral result of this form of parental "attention" is decreased withdrawal, less insistent protest and defensiveness, and increased compliance with parental demands (Parpal and Maccoby, 1985). It is also likely that this form of engagement between parent and child strengthens a less observable, but still essential, process: that a parent's affirming responsiveness helps preserve the child's admiration for her parent, a cornerstone of successful socialization and the development of a moral self.

And there are other benefits as well. The child accrues, in the course of these playful interactions, some increment in her capacity to tolerate frustrations and disappointments (Chapter 9). Something will not go the way the child wants it to go—for example, the blocks will fall down—and the parent is there, to offer consolation and to help the child find some alternative, through their combined ingenuity and imagination. If she doesn't have the block that she needs or wants, perhaps she can use this one instead. The child learns, in these moments, that disappointments are temporary, that frustrations can be "handled," and that problems can be solved (and that it cannot always be her way). She has also learned, in a small way, to make accommodations to others, a social skill essential for successful peer relationships.

Greenspan's Floor Time program (see, especially, Greenspan and Wieder, 1998) provides a paradigm for this kind of parent-child interaction. I therefore recommend—to all families—some adaptation of Floor Time, appropriate to the age, temperament, and developmental level of the child. Floor Time procedures, developed as a therapeutic intervention for children with profound deficits in social engagement, are beneficial for all children. In my experience, both in my general out-patient practice and in interviews of children hospitalized for severe aggressive behavior, even deeply suspicious and defiant children continue to seek—and respond favorably—to this form of affirming interaction.

Many concerned and caring parents, for reasons of personality or life circumstance, find it difficult to engage with their children in this way—they may tell us that they lack the time or the interest. But we should not give up. If we are able to help parents find opportunities for more frequent play and playfulness with their children, the parents will be rewarded—with increased pleasure in being a parent. And the child, sensing the parent's pleasure, will more often and more eagerly seek out this engagement. In this way, we set in motion a cycle of *positive* interactions that begins to reverse the *vicious* cycles of criticism and defiance that are so prevalent in the lives of troubled families.

As with any therapeutic intervention, of course, we cannot be certain how far the therapeutic benefit of these interactions extends. We do not know to what extent high "doses" of shared interest and interactive play can ameliorate the symptoms of withdrawal and defiance in children of different ages. It may be helpful to think of positive affect sharing and responsive play as the psychological equivalent of good nutrition. Nutrition does not prevent all diseases or cure disease processes once they have reached a certain stage of development. Still, good psychological nutrition is essential to the emotional health of the child and helps promote psychological immunity. And we know that these moments are important in the lives of children—because children tell us about them. Considering the undeniable benefits of these interactions: increased pleasure, improved compliance, and the strengthening of social skills, there is no reason not to make interactive play a first recommendation or "prescription" for parents of almost all children.[5]

Criticism

If I were asked to identify the most common problem presented to me in three decades of clinical work with children and families, my answer would be unequivocal: "As parents, we are, unwittingly, too critical of our children." Research findings reported by John Gottman and his colleagues now provide empirical support for this anecdotal claim. Gottman, Katz, and Hooven (1997) offer compelling evidence of the harmful effects of parental criticism (what Gottman calls "derogation") on children's emotions, academic achievement, peer relations, and physiology, including increased production of stress-related hormones that are potentially damaging to brain development. In these studies of parent-child communication, the parental behavior most directly related to measurable physiological stress in children was derogation or mockery, especially, by fathers (Gottman, 1997; Gottman, Katz, and Hooven, 1997).[6]

Every parental criticism evokes in the child a complex emotional response. The child's response to criticism generally includes both some degree of demoralization and, even more regularly, a defiant-retaliatory reaction, expressed as defensiveness or argument (often as inner argument) and then, increasingly, as grievance. I have come to regard this sequence of events, with some exaggeration, as the psychological equivalent of Newton's Third Law: Every parental criticism evokes in the child an equal and opposite defiant reaction. As in physics, the nature of the opposing reaction (i.e., the child's defiant response) depends upon other forces that are present (i.e., the child's temperament and personality) and may not be openly expressed or immediately observable. Persistent criticism, however, breeds demoralization, resentment, and defiance and is therefore profoundly destructive of the child's initiative and self-confidence. We need to prevent the further build-up of these damaging attitudes in the mind of the child.

We all know, from our own lives, how criticism feels. We may have experienced the demoralizing effect of frequent criticism (or the mere absence of praise, appreciation, and other forms of recognition) in the work place, or the eroding effect of frequent criticism on satisfaction in love relationships. It is surprising, then, how frequently we fail to consider this in relation to our children. Many families are unaware of the presence of this toxin. Criticism has become part of the family atmosphere, undetected or accepted as "normal" to those inside the family, but immediately apparent to an outside observer.[7] In still other families, parents feel justified in their criticism—and children, for their part, feel increasingly justified in their resentment and defiance. Parents tell us that, "He never listens." The child tells us, "All I hear is criticism" or "They are always yelling at me."

It seems necessary to ask, and I have often discussed with colleagues, "Why are parents so often critical of their children?" It is inevitable, of course, that parents will criticize their children. Criticism from parents and teachers (optimally, in my opinion, in small doses and "sandwiched" between encouragement and praise for increments of effort and success) is a necessary part of learning. Much parental criticism is well-intentioned, motivated by a parent's desire for the child to "improve" and eventually succeed in a competitive world. In these instances, parents criticize because they are anxious about the child's future. They regard their criticism as "constructive," or not as criticism at all, but rather as instruction. Parents feel especially justified in their criticism when the child's misbehavior is egregious, and when they make an effort to balance criticism with praise. Because they are willing to offer praise for the child's good behavior, these parents do not regard themselves as critical.

Some parents have expressed the opinion that it is their "right and responsibility" to be critical of their children—to tell the child what she is doing wrong—in order to prepare her for the demands and responsibilities she will face as an adult. In a sense, these parents are right—some form of guidance and instruction, both practical and moral, is essential to the successful socialization of the child. From this perspective, shared by many clinicians, the child's defiance (or withdrawal, or unwillingness to communicate), especially in adolescence, is a normal consequence of responsible parenting. I question this assumption. It is, of course, true that parents often must express disapproval and say, "No" to their children, and that children can be expected to respond with some form of protest when limits are set. Persistent criticism, however, damages parent-child relationships and a "balance," or equal ratio, of praise and criticism is far from optimal.[8]

Finally, many parents are critical because the child's feelings or behavior evokes their own unacknowledged resentments and disappointments—their own bad feelings. And, often, they do not know another way.

In families where pathogenic cycles of criticism and defiance are present, it is essential to educate parents about the destructive effects of persistent criticism and to help parents find an alternative—to begin to replace criticism with inquiry, understanding, and problem-solving. In my personal and supervisory experience, a therapist's failure to identify and alleviate persistent (albeit often unwitting) criticism undermines all other therapeutic efforts and is a common source of therapeutic failure or, at least, limits the success of all other therapeutic interventions.

When parents are angry and critical with their children, children, in turn, become angry and argumentative, stubborn and defiant. And parents who argue frequently with their children beget children who are good at arguing—or children who give up, and then continue the argument silently.

Repair

We need to offer these families a way out—a way to arrest vicious cycles of criticism and defiance, to replace criticism with understanding and appreciation. This is a critical therapeutic process for many families, especially when argument and opposition have developed extensively and become habitual. The antidotes to criticism—simple in theory, but difficult in practice—are patient listening, recognition of the child's efforts, praise for small increments of pro-social behavior, and a proactive approach to ameliorating recurrent problematic situations.

We begin, as always, with an empathic understanding of the parents' concerns. In my experience, the *proximate* cause of most parental criticism is a parent's anxiety and frustration—most often, anxiety about the child's welfare, in the present and, especially, in the future. (The *ultimate* causes of persistent criticism are rooted in the parent's character and life circumstances, how well the parent copes with painful feelings in his own life, and how burdened the parent feels by the demands of raising children.) A working class father, frustrated by his son's poor grades and inconsistent effort at schoolwork, asks, in frustration, "Do you want to end up like me, collecting coins from parking meters?"

We need to help parents find ways to listen more patiently to the child's concerns and grievances—*to understand what is important to the child*—and then to replace criticism, in whatever way possible, with encouragement and praise. There is no better antidote for frequent criticism and argument—and no better way to help children bounce back from the common frustrations and disappointments of childhood—than patient and respectful listening (Nichols, 2004). Listening, of course, does not mean agreement or giving in to unreasonable demands, but rather, making some effort to understand and appreciate the child's point of view, and to acknowledge what is *right* about what the child is saying before we point out what is *wrong*.

In therapeutic work with families, we help parents create moments that are conducive to this kind of patient listening, not only in therapy sessions, but also in daily family life. For many families, I recommend that parents set aside some extra time, perhaps 10 minutes at bedtime, as a time for the child to have a chance to talk. In these brief daily conversations, the child is encouraged to say whatever she was upset or angry about during the day, or to talk about what she liked (and didn't like), or what she may be anxious about the following day. And when the child has nothing to talk about, parents can make use of this opportunity to talk about the events of their day, perhaps to share a frustration or a moment of humor. Children look forward to these moments, just as they do opportunities to play. It is surprising, then, how infrequently families make this a regular part of the child's day. Often, when parents regularly put aside time to listen and talk with their children, they report immediate improvement in the child's mood and behavior.

These are also moments when parents may be able to *initiate* repair. In every family—but more often in troubled families—parents, when they are anxious and frustrated, will become harshly critical and may say hurtful things to their children. At these times, it is important for us to help parents initiate reparative experiences.[9] Parents should acknowledge their errors, reestablish dialogue, and, when appropriate, frankly apologize to their child.

I encourage parents to find a time when the child is likely to be receptive, to "take responsibility" for their own emotional response (to say to the child, for example, "I know I was very angry at you earlier. Maybe I got *too* angry"), and to make some effort to appreciate, or at least acknowledge, the child's point of view ("I know you really wanted to…"). Some parents express concern that, in apologizing to their children, they may implicitly sanction the child's behavior and diminish their authority as parents. A parental apology, however, does not excuse a child's bad behavior ("You still should not have hit your sister"). And understanding a child's mood is not the same as indulging a child's mood; the needs of others always have to be considered. In my opinion, when a parent initiates repair and offers an apology, he has modeled an important lesson in interpersonal relationships and *gains* authority with his child—because the child's acceptance of adult authority is ultimately based on respect.

When listening to a child's grievance, I encourage parents to *simply listen*; discussion and disagreement can come later. Optimally, the parent should approach the child with modesty and respect ("I want to understand better how you feel") and a genuine desire to find ways to alleviate the child's distress. And it is important to give the child time—the parent should not, at that moment, insist on a response. Many clinicians have noted (see, for example, Kindlon and Thompson, 1999; Pollack, 1998) that this may be especially important for boys, who often need more time to let go of their reflexive defensiveness.

At the end of the day, we have no substitute for and no better "techniques" to promote resilience than joyful play and patient listening. Often, this is all that is necessary. And we should certainly count as a therapeutic success, when a child tells us, "I don't have to come here any more. Now I'm having good talks with my mom."

Proactive Problem-solving

Even after successful reparative moments, however, there is still a problem—often, a recurring problem. The child may have lied, been disrespectful, refused to cooperate, or failed to do his homework. And actions have consequences; some punishment may be necessary. Recurring problematic moments in the life of the child and family are best solved—and perhaps can *only* be solved—proactively. Parents who are *re-acting* to their child's behavior will often be reacting badly.

A proactive approach to problem-solving consists of several elements:

(1) Identify recurrent problematic situations. Parents should say to the child, for example, "We have a problem in the mornings, when it's time to get ready, and I often end up yelling at you" or "A lot of times, we have a problem when I tell you that it is time to turn off the television."

(2) Communicate some appreciation of the problem from the child's point of view. It is especially important to acknowledge the child's grievance—what the child believes is unfair and *why this is important to the child.*

(3) Elicit the child's ideas. It seems almost reflexive for many parents, when faced with a child's persistent defiance or lack of cooperation, to attempt to solve these problems by imposing a "consequence" for the child's misbehavior. Although some problems may require this approach, I recommend that parents first engage the child in an effort to solve the problem—to elicit the child's ideas. In this way (as with Julia, in Chapter 2), we are often able to engage the child in a search for solutions. The child is then less absorbed in angry, defiant modes of thought, in making demands or continuing the argument.

Listening to the child's ideas does not diminish a parent's authority. Parents retain their authority to establish rules and consequences, and there are many situations, especially those that involve safety and the rights of others, when rules are explained, but are not negotiable.

(4) Help the child develop explicit emotion-regulation strategies—what the child can *do* when she is angry or upset. Cognitive-behavioral treatments for children and adolescents emphasize this step in the problem-solving process and have contributed valuable techniques that help both parents and children reduce urgent feelings of anxiety, anger, and emotional distress (see, for example, Kendall, Aschenbrand, and Hudson, 2003 and Kendall and Suveg, 2006, on techniques to help children manage anxiety; Seligman, 1995 and Stark et al., 2008, on strategies to combat pessimistic thinking and support assertive problem-solving; Lochman et al., 2006, on a cognitive approach to reducing aggressive behavior in children; and Nelson, Finch, and Ghee, 2006, on cognitive-behavioral techniques for "anger management"). These "cognitive-behavioral" strategies are emotion-regulation strategies. The child learns how thinking influences feeling, and that there is more than one way

to solve a problem and to feel better. Many children, especially if we have prepared them with an appreciation of their needs and concerns, participate enthusiastically in this process. The child may make a list of "things I can do when I'm upset" (for example, draw, write, or play with her dolls). Or, for a young child who is angry, we can suggest that she go to an "angry spot" in her room. Or, a child might ask a parent to use a signal, a word that the parent can invoke as a warning to the child that her language or behavior is "over the line."

However, if a parent has not first listened to the child's grievance, the child is likely to be a half-hearted participant in this problem-solving process, and any strategies we offer to help the child regulate her emotions are likely to be ineffective. In my experience, these techniques are also unlikely to be helpful once the child's distress or anger has passed a certain threshold. Children often tell us that they cannot make us of these techniques, even when they would like to, when they are "too angry"; and we have known for a long time that once a tantrum has started, most often, it has to run its course (Parens, 1987).

(5) Parents then need to offer praise—expressions of appreciation and recognition—for every increment of the child's effort at compliance and self-control. Many parents neglect this essential step. The child's efforts at self-control are too quickly taken for granted and, following some initial improvement, the family tells us that the plan "did not work"—that they are back to square one.

(6) Parents also need to establish rules and enforce consequences (punishments) for persistent or egregious violations of these rules. Children understand this—all families have rules.[10] Many children, especially younger children, also benefit from a simple incentive program—earning tangible rewards—for compliance with rules and for pro-social behavior. I will discuss the problem of establishing family rules and limits in greater detail in the following chapter.

Again, Sharings

Young children are wide-eyed in their curiosity about the lives of their parents. For many years, I have advised parents to talk with their children about experiences in their own lives, especially at times of sadness, anxiety, or disappointment—the child's anxiety, for example, about her first day at school or summer camp, or an upcoming exam; a painful rejection by a friend; difficulties in school; or a death in the family. Telling personal stories to children—and in the presence of children—is an important socialization practice in many cultures. (Often, these are cautionary tales, of dangers to avoid—or of virtues to be admired). Personal sharings offer hope to an anxious or discouraged child.

In my experience, there simply is no better way, as a parent or therapist, to engage a young child's attention and provide emotional support than these, essentially humanizing, personal disclosures.[11]

A First and Final Principle: Staying Positive

There is a frequently cited rule among those who sell real estate, that the value of any property is determined by three factors: location, location, and location. In my opinion, there is an equivalent rule for parents and child therapists in promoting emotional resilience in children: be positive, be positive, be positive. This is a first and final principle of helping parents help their children, perhaps more important than any other.

Most parents would agree with this primary parental function, that children are likely to thrive when parents are supportive and encouraging, and nurture in their children a positive future orientation. In the daily life of many families, however, moments of encouragement and affirmation have become infrequent, and "parenting"[12] descends into taxiing the child to and from her various activities and making sure that she has done her homework or cleaned her room. It is disheartening to observe how often caring parents have become preoccupied with their child's misbehavior and overlook opportunities to express appreciation and praise. Expressions of appreciation, small and large, are essential in all love and work relationships, including parent-child relationships.

Parents can remain positive with their children by making note of each increment in the child's effort and pro-social behavior. They will then find many more occasions for the expression of confidence and pride. We should also encourage parents to offer opportunities for their children to earn appreciation—for carrying out responsibilities at home and at school, and for helping others (for example, reading to a younger child)—and to provide, on a daily basis, some affirming experience, perhaps a shared meal or prayer.

Wachtel (2001) has wisely advised that parents should cultivate, in talking with their children, "a language of becoming"—"a way of speaking to children that enables them to see themselves as continually evolving and changing" (p. 369) and "as developing emotional strengths" (p. 372). A language of becoming allows parents to notice the child's "new actions" and focus on what is positive and hopeful, rather than problematic, in the child's behavior. Wachtel notes, for example, that "when a child has had an explosive episode but eventually calms himself down and talks about the problem more rationally, a parent has the choice of focusing either on the explosion or on how the youngster was able to calm himself down enough to have a rational discussion about the problem" (p. 372).

Wachtel also reminds us of other affirming experiences—moments in our lives that may be of lasting importance. "Most of us have had at one time or another the experience of being 'discovered.' Perhaps it was a visiting aunt, or a teacher, or a boyfriend who saw in us something that transformed—or at least greatly influenced—how we saw ourselves. Many people can remember a compliment, comment, or reflection on themselves that stuck with them for the rest of their lives . . . These statements can serve as emotional life preservers in stormy seas" (p. 371). Wachtel is correct in making note of the importance of these moments in the life of the child. I recommend her article as a "must read" for all child therapists.

Bobby: Refusal

Many of the concerns presented to us by parents are expressions of defiance and refusal. Bobby, a 9-year-old boy, refused to turn off the television, or to brush his teeth; he often refused to eat, but he would later sneak candy into his room. He refused to do his homework, then refused to go to school, setting in motion the "power struggles" so common in contemporary family life. In Bobby's family, these "battles" took an increasingly malignant form.

Mr. N.: "If you don't turn off the television (or stop playing Game Boy), you will not have a play date tomorrow."

Bobby ignores his father.

Mr. N. repeats and increases his threat, ". . . or the next day."

Bobby continues to ignore his father.

Mr. N. turns off the television. Bobby begins hitting his father, throwing the remote control, and threatens to kill his parents or kill himself. He goes into his bedroom, throwing objects and ripping posters off the wall (or, on other occasions, he would lie motionless on the floor). Mr. N. attempts to restrain Bobby from throwing things by holding him down.

Bobby continues to fight.

Mr. N., in desperation, calls the police.

Bobby's refusals were often sudden, unexpected, and unpredictable. If he had difficulty doing his homework, he would often give up, refuse to work, then refuse to go to school the next day. He might also refuse to go to school if he had been angry at his parents the night before, but not always. He refused to go on a class trip. His parents and therapist wondered if he might be anxious about the bus ride; does he feel excluded, or even bullied? But Bobby refused to give any explanation. Bobby told his therapist, "Yes, there is something" he was anxious about, but he would not say what it was.

Over the past two years, Bobby's relationship with his father had deteriorated. Bobby and Mr. N. now spent very little time together, and Bobby seemed to harbor a deep grievance against his father. Mr. N., who cared deeply about his son, had become increasingly frustrated and angry. He was critical of his wife's "indulgence"—certain that Bobby was spoiled and that his wife was at fault.

Bobby was a good student. Although he often did not complete his homework, Bobby's teachers were pleased with his contributions in class.

Neuropsychological evaluation had revealed no evidence of an attention or learning disorder. Bobby would immediately give up, however, when his schoolwork became difficult. He told his parents, "I must be stupid" and he was resistant to instruction of all kinds. In rare moments of openness, Bobby complained, "I'm always unhappy."

How had these behavioral and emotional problems developed? Why did Bobby so insistently respond to any anxiety or frustration with intransigent refusal? Bobby's parents disagreed; increasingly, Mr. and Mrs. N. seemed pushed into polar attitudes toward Bobby's behavior. Mr. N. believed that Bobby was "getting away with it," that his demands had "worked." And, at least to some extent, this was true: Bobby could coerce his mother, by threatening a tantrum, into extending his playtime, and he had become practiced at bribes and threats. ("If you don't buy me a new baseball bat now, I won't go to school," or even, "If you don't buy me ice cream, I won't put on my seatbelt.") Mrs. N. believed that Bobby's father was at fault: "You are too harsh with him...you are making him more angry and defiant." And this was also true.

The previous year, Mrs. N. had been seriously ill, requiring a lengthy period of hospitalization. Both Mr. and Mrs. N. wondered about the impact of this event on Bobby's mood and behavior. From early childhood, Bobby had had difficulty making friends; although not ostracized, he now often compared himself unfavorably to his peers. To what extent did anxiety about peer relationships contribute to Bobby's refusals?

As is often the case, the causes of Bobby's difficulties remained obscure. Over time, however, Bobby had developed a defiant and coercive—as opposed to a resilient or problem-solving—mode of coping with frustration and anxiety. Bobby had become stubborn and uncommunicative, and his family relationships were increasingly troubled, stuck in a vicious cycle of anger and defiance.

As a supervisor of Bobby's therapist, I recommended a multidimensional approach to treatment, including consultation with Bobby's teachers. Medicine had been prescribed, with little apparent benefit, and was discontinued. Bobby talked easily with his therapist, a warm and empathic young woman who was, in fact, easy to talk with. Bobby talked with Dr. L. especially about his interests, including interests they shared (for example, science) and if Bobby was interested in something Dr. L. knew little about (for example, Pokemon and baseball), he was happy to teach her. He enjoyed playing games and created "tournaments" between himself and Dr. L., which he was almost always able to win. If he lost, he gave up that competition and created a new tournament, with a different game. (Bobby told Dr. L., "I used to play checkers with my dad, but he beat me, so I stopped playing.")

But Bobby would not talk about why he was angry or why he wouldn't go to school. On these matters, it seemed that Bobby had taken a vow of silence. "When I talk about being angry, he explained to Dr. L., it just makes me more angry." It is likely that Bobby's refusal to talk included many of the elements that commonly comprise a child's resistance: not talking had become Bobby's habitual mode of coping with distress and part of his ongoing protest and argument; he was also afraid that talking about bad feelings wouldn't help, that he would just feel bad all over again—and this may have been the core of Bobby's resistance.

Dr. L. met frequently with Bobby's parents—to help Mr. and Mrs. N. come together and establish some common understanding about how to respond to Bobby's refusals, and to find ways to effect some repair of parent-child relationships, especially Bobby's relationship with his father. Anger, disappointment, argument, and defiance had eroded away most emotional sharing in this father-son relationship. First, father and son began to spend time together, playing soccer in the back yard; then, at a later time, Mr. N. initiated some discussion—an effort at repair of angry moments, as much as Bobby would allow. Often, the best Mr. N. could do was to indicate his willingness to talk, but Bobby refused.

Mr. and Mrs. N. also needed a plan. How should they respond to major and minor problems of daily compliance, when Bobby refused to turn off the television, refused to do his homework, or refused to go to school? How could they avoid escalating threats and physical confrontations? Bobby's parents asked for guidance: what should they do if Bobby woke up in the morning and said, "I'm not going to school?"

I recommended to Dr. L. that Mr. and Mrs. N. should engage Bobby in the solution of recurrent problems. Bobby's proposals (for example, "Let me stay up as late as I want") were often unacceptable (and still somewhat in the nature of a threat or a demand) but, at least, he had begun to consider a solution. Like many children, Bobby often said that he "didn't care" about punishments or consequences. If he wasn't allowed to go the movies, or play with a friend, or watch television, or use the computer, he would just stay home and read (and he was sure that they would never take away his books). But of course, he *did* care. Mr. and Mrs. N. established a straightforward system of basic responsibilities, with rewards and "consequences" (i.e., punishments—no electronics if he is at home; no weekend play dates), especially if Bobby refused to go to school. And Bobby could earn things he wanted by doing his homework and basic chores.

Slowly, there were signs of progress. In some unguarded moments, Bobby began to talk, tentatively (as we all do about things we feel badly about), in a way that might feel somewhat less shameful. With his therapist—and with his parents—Bobby began to talk about difficulties with his friends and (hypothetically) about "how to get people to do what they don't want to do." (Bobby offered his solution to this problem: "Bribe them . . . or trick them.") He was willing to try new activities—Little League and Cub Scouts. The anxiety that preceded Bobby's refusals now became more apparent; when he was frustrated or upset, he would no longer break things, but would begin to cry.

There are many ways to understand the process of change, many explanations of how Bobby was able emerge from a persistent pattern of defiance and refusal. Although he could still become stubborn and demanding, in a little over a year since his beginning therapy, Bobby was now a generally happy, normally functioning boy. It could be argued that Bobby had responded favorably to a more consistent exercise of parental authority, that through firm and reasonable enforcement of rewards and punishments, Mr. and Mrs. N. had been able to diminish coercive patterns of family interactions; in this way, Bobby had learned that demands and refusal no longer "worked," forcing him to develop more mature behaviors when he was frustrated and angry. Bobby's discussions—and his play—with Dr. L. seemed to have helped him, gradually, to "open up"—to risk the expression of unpleasant feelings and to respond with less stubbornness when things did not go his way. As Dr. L. and I tried to understand these changes together, however, we sensed that the crucial change in Bobby's life was the repair of his relationship with his father. Bobby and Mr. N. now enjoyed many activities together and Bobby looked forward to spending time with his dad. A vicious cycle of anger, defiance, and grievance in this father-son relationship had been arrested and then reversed. This change, we believed, more than any other, allowed Bobby to bounce back from moments of refusal and to approach the opportunities and challenges in his life with greater willingness and enthusiasm.

Notes

1. Gottman, Katz, and Hooven (1997) report a search of the popular literature on parent guidance. This search yielded "1412 references on 'parent and discipline' and 69 references on 'parent and emotion.'" Gottman, Katz, and Hooven note that "most parenting guides address themselves to parents who feel out of control, to those whose major issue is obtaining compliance, obedience, and respect from their children" (p. 14).

   There are important exceptions to this trend. Many excellent programs have been developed for professionals that approach parent guidance with the fundamental, and I believe ultimately more important, goal of improving parent-child relationships. Cavell (2000) has presented a model of working with parents of aggressive children based on helping parents promote in their children a sense of "acceptance" and "containment," in conjunction with the parents' consistent endorsement and modeling of pro-social values.

   Greene and Ablon's (2006) collaborative problem-solving (CPS) approach to the treatment of "explosive" children deserves special mention. Greene and Ablon regard compliance ("defined as the capacity to defer or delay one's own goals in response to the imposed goals or standards of an authority figure") as "one of many developmental expressions of the skills of flexibility/adaptability, frustration tolerance, and problem solving in young children" (p. 8). Noncompliance reflects a delay in the development of these skills. In the Greene and Ablon model, collaborative problem-solving begins with empathy—an explicit recognition of the concerns of both children and parents. Therapists then help parents "identify the triggers that precipitate explosive episodes" (p. 52). In this way, the child's explosive behavior becomes "highly predictable" and the triggers for these episodes are understood as "problems to be solved." Parents are helped to become "a surrogate frontal lobe" for their children, "modeling and teaching the crucial skills of flexibility, frustration tolerance, and problem solving" (p. 52). The CPS model is, in its essentials, identical to the proactive problem-solving component of the approach to parent guidance I recommend in this chapter.

Other exceptions to the behavioral emphasis of advice to parents are approaches to parent guidance based on attachment theory, with the goal of facilitating increased parental insightfulness (Koren-Karie, Oppenheim, and Goldsmith, 2007), mentalization (Bleiberg, Fonagy, and Target, 1997), and reflective functioning (Slade, 2006).

Among books addressed to the general public, I would note, especially, Greenspan (1993; 1995), Gottman (1997), Nichols (2004), Siegel and Hartzell (2003), Marston (1990), and Ginott's (1965) classic, *Between Parent and Child.*

2. These are most often, although not always, our concerns as well. In the early years of my practice, I was consulted by the affluent parents of a withdrawn and oppositional 12-year-old boy. I met with this boy for several sessions, and I believed he was deeply troubled—angry and unhappy. His parents, however, saw only his lack of effort and initiative with regard to schoolwork. Among the parents' complaints was the boy's insufficient effort at practicing the saxophone, which they expected, already at this age, would help pay his way through college. Knowing, even as I spoke, that my comment was probably ill-timed and unwise, I suggested that perhaps he should play music simply for the enjoyment of playing. The parents terminated the boy's therapy shortly thereafter, with the brief explanation that they believed I was too much on "the child's side" and they sought out a different therapist. I don't know if I would be able to respond differently today. Clearly, this is the most difficult aspect of our work—the task of understanding, but also effectively challenging, parents whose values are different from our own, parents, for example, who feel entirely justified in their punitiveness toward their children; or who believe in a degree of "toughness" that we believe is destructive; parents who do not seem interested in spending time with their children; or parents who believe, as one mother recently told me, that "childhood is not a time to have fun."
3. Granic and Patterson (2006), from the perspective of dynamic systems theory, make the important observation that the emotional landscape of almost all families is characterized by "multistability," that is, angry and critical interactions are not the only "attractors" that exert gravitational pull in a family.
4. Cavell (2000) advises that therapists can strengthen their alliance with families—and learn more about what it is like to be a parent of an aggressive child—by simply "letting parents tell their story." And Greene and Ablon (2006) make the important clinical observation that, when describing their child's explosive behavior, parents "need to be *believed*" (p. 22). It is easy to forget these elementary therapeutic principles in our zeal to promote positive changes in a parent's behavior. To be frank, as I review my own work with families over the past several years, when I have been unsuccessful in helping families—or when promising beginnings have ended prematurely—it is almost always at this step that I have gone wrong.

5. Greenspan and Wieder (1997) report encouraging preliminary empirical support for Floor Time as a therapeutic intervention for children with autistic spectrum disorders, based on a chart review. Fifty-eight percent of autistic children who received the Floor Time treatment program showed "good to outstanding" improvement. Greenspan (1993; 1995) has also recommended Floor Time as an essential component of "healthy parenting."

   We should note an important convergence of different theoretical perspectives in recommending responsive play between parents and children. In addition to Greenspan's Floor Time program, responsive play is an important element of the treatment program developed by Webster-Stratton and Reid (2003) and of Barkley's (1997b) behavioral program for defiant children.
6. Webster-Stratton and Reid (2003), in a 12-year follow-up of families who received the Incredible Years family treatment program, report that a mother's level of criticism and a father's use of praise were important predictors of adjustment in adolescence. In a separate evaluation of a child-focused Incredible Years intervention program, children whose parents continued to use high levels of criticism and physical spankings derived the least benefit from the treatment. See also Alloy et al., 2001, from the perspective of cognitive theory, on the role of parental criticism ("negative inferential feedback") in the vulnerability to depression in late adolescence.
7. Many years ago, because no seats were available in nonsmoking cars, I was forced to sit in the smoking car of a commuter train. As I entered the car, a thick cloud of smoke was immediately visible. After a short time, however, I no longer saw the pollution that was so apparent just a few minutes before; it was now "normal." When my eyes began to tear, I briefly wondered why this was happening. A toxin that had becomes invisible was, of course, still able to produce symptoms. This is what criticism is like in many families.
8. An equal ratio of praise and criticism has been shown to be unhealthy, both in marriage (Gottman, 1994) and in parent-child relationships (Kazdin, 2005).
9. Seigel and Hartzell (2003) refer to this as the "repair of toxic ruptures."
10. A defiant adolescent may insist that all rules and restrictions are coercive and espouse, instead, a crude philosophy of anarchism. But, even then, if we listen with enough patience and respect, she is likely to soften this defiant attitude and admit that, perhaps, not all laws are unjust.
11. I learned the value of telling personal stories as a young parent. Our daughter, Rachel, was not yet 3 years old when our son, Dan, was born. The new baby slept in a bassinet in our bedroom for a few months until it was time for him to share a bedroom with his sister. Until now, Rachel had seemed pleased with her new role as a big sister and had expressed little jealousy of her baby brother. But this night, when going to bed, she told me, "I don't want my baby brother sleeping in my room." This, I thought, would be an easy problem to solve, a piece of cake. I was, after all, a child psychologist and this was Child Psych 101. I told Rachel that I could understand her feelings. We were able to give her less attention than before the baby was born. And this room used to be *her* room—now, it was *the children's* room. Rachel listened to my sympathetic explanations and, when I had finished, she replied, "Well, that's OK, but I still don't want my baby brother sleeping in my room." Not knowing what else to do, I offered a personal story. "Let me tell you about when daddy was a little

boy and I slept in the same room with Uncle Bob and Uncle Steve." Rachel's eyes widened. To this point, she had listened with polite attention; now, she listened with rapt attention. I told her a (true) story about sharing a room with my brothers and she quickly fell asleep. Then, the following night and for several months thereafter, as I put her to bed, she asked, "Tell me a story about when you were a little boy."

12. If I may be allowed a bit of crankiness: this common usage—"parenting" as a verb—implicitly diminishes what may be most essential about being a parent, as if being a parent can be reduced to a set of rules or behavioral "techniques." Parents' words and actions toward their children are, of course, important, and, in most instances, they are the appropriate focus of therapeutic work. But there are also less tangible ways in which parents are important to their children, behaviors that preserve the child's respect for her parents and her confident expectation of parental support, and that convince the child that her parents still "count." (Recall Erikson's statement that a secure sense of identity depends on "the assuredness of anticipated recognition from those who count.") Children come to understand the character of their parents, how parents cope with conflict and adversity, and they observe how parents treat each other. We learn, sadly, from helping children who have witnessed severe marital conflict or an adversarial divorce, that the denigration of either parent may have a profoundly destructive effect on children, leading to disillusionment and cynicism, regardless of a parent's otherwise appropriate "parenting" skills.

12

Parent Guidance II: Helping Parents with Common Problems of Daily Living

Parents present us with many concerns about their children. They may initially seek consultation and treatment because of a child's aggressive behavior or difficulty making friends. But, in the course of our work, other problems are regularly brought to our attention: a child's difficulty falling asleep at night; fighting with siblings; and battles over chores, homework, and, increasingly, television and electronic games. For these common concerns, many parents ask our "expert" guidance; often, they have "tried everything."

In this chapter, I will offer strategies to help families resolve or ameliorate many of these common, yet often intractable, problems of daily living. These recommendations are informed by the same basic principle that underlies all of our therapeutic efforts: we help children learn, in manageable increments, to tolerate—and then bounce back from—the anxieties, frustrations, and disappointments that occur, on a daily basis, in childhood and throughout life.

First, however, a caveat: The solution of almost all common problems of childhood should not be attempted piecemeal. Every problematic behavior presented to us by parents requires detailed inquiry and an assessment of its possible causes. And these problems of daily living will be resolved more quickly and more successfully when parents have been able to put into practice the principles of emotional health and resilience discussed in the previous chapter—empathic understanding, responsive play, repair of angry and critical interactions, a proactive approach to problem-solving, encouragement and support. A family atmosphere of frequent argument, resentment, and withdrawal undermines our best efforts to solve any common problem.

Rules and Limits

The problem of behavioral compliance—"he never listens"—remains the overriding concern of modern parents. Behavioral limits, of course, are necessary in the socialization of all children. In previous chapters, I discussed what I believe are the fundamental processes of successful socialization and moral development—parental responsiveness, interactive play, and the internalization of parental pride. I presented the thesis that children most effectively learn behavioral limits in the context of pleasurable, interactive play with an admired adult who makes implicit and explicit behavioral demands. In these interactions, the child comes to understand and accept, deeply and for the right reasons, that rules are necessary—for safety and for living with others. In my opinion, therefore, a narrow focus on compliant behavior—how parents should "set limits" for their children—is rarely, as therapists, our most important concern.

Parents, however, ask for—and need—behavioral advice. And, as proponents of behavioral methods have correctly pointed out, for many families, the implementation of a successful program to promote compliant behavior is an important step toward creating a more affirming family environment. Increased compliance relieves parents of daily sources of frustration and resentment, allowing them to then engage more positively with their children—and with each other.

Successful behavioral programs for children with oppositional behavior and disorders of conduct have been developed and tested. Principles derived from these programs—although based on theoretical premises that are different from my own—can be readily incorporated into a comprehensive treatment plan. Kazdin (2005) reports significant advances in our understanding of the essential elements of effective behavioral interventions for children. Parents (and teachers) need to understand these basic principles: (1) the importance of *frequent praise* (reinforcement) for *small increments* of compliance, pro-social behavior, and efforts at behavioral control (for example, waiting) and (2) the need to be judicious in the use of punishment. As praise has increasingly taken precedence over punishment (or "consequences") in contemporary behavior management programs, distinctions between behaviorist and non-behaviorist approaches to child discipline have waned. Behavioral and emotion-focused clinicians can now find more common ground.[1]

What follows is a general framework for establishing family rules and enforcing behavioral limits that has been helpful to many parents. In these few pages, I cannot address all of the problematic situations parents face in making disciplinary decisions about their children; there are too many difficult situations, each involving questions of degree. And, in any difficult moment, when a parent asks, "Does this behavior merit a punishment, or is it better to let this one go?" there may not be a "correct" answer. We can provide guidelines, but not a script. Parental decisions about how to respond to a child's challenging behavior always involve listening and judgment, and some effort to balance empathy and firmness. Our ultimate goal is to help the child develop discipline in the best sense—the ability to forgo immediate pleasure, or to endure frustration, in the service of long-term goals. And it is helpful for parents—especially parents who frequently disagree—to realize that each parental decision about a child's behavior is not critical. It is more important that parents:

(1) establish some reasonable limits—so that the child comes to understand the need for limits,

(2) avoid "escalations" and "negative reciprocity" (Forgatch, Bullock, and Patterson, 2004)—vicious cycles of negative interactions that breed defiance, resentment, and despair,

(3) understand that criticism is hurtful, and

(4) that expressions of encouragement and appreciation are vital. These moments "stay with" the child and help children sustain a positive future orientation.

If we have been able to help parents create a more positive family atmosphere—an atmosphere in which children look forward to spending time with their parents and are willing to share their concerns, at least some of the time—the problem of setting limits will be far easier. (Although, admittedly, especially for impulsive or hyperactive children, it is not always easy.) In families with little positive engagement and supportive listening, parents' attempts to set limits are likely to be difficult and often unsuccessful, complicated by the child's covert defiance and opposition.

In helping parents set rules and limits for their children, I suggest to parents that almost all non-negotiable rules fall into two basic categories:

(1) *to protect the child's health and safety* (for example, the child must always wear a seatbelt, or a helmet when riding a bicycle) and

(2) *to respect the rights of others* (for example, the child's language may not be hurtful or abusive, and his brother or sister must also get a turn).[2]

These restrictions on the child's freedom are easily understood—and readily accepted—by most children. I recommend these guidelines, especially, for parents who are uncertain about what "battles" to choose—what rules to strictly enforce and when to allow the child greater freedom of choice and expression.

Parents then establish a few simple family rules. A basic rule for all children is a limit on physical and verbal aggression. For younger children: no hitting, no screaming, no bad words, and cooperate with parents, especially during recurring problematic moments (for example, getting ready in the morning or going to bed on time). The same rules apply to older children, with perhaps some others (for example, limits on the use electronic games and helping with basic household chores). The simplicity of family rules is important—simple rules are unarguable (most of the time) and therefore more effectively enforced.

In talking with children, I have found it helpful to emphasize the obviousness of a family's need for rules ("Of course, kids need to have a bed time" or "I never heard of a kid who could watch TV *all day*"). And, although the child may briefly protest, kids get it. (This is especially true before defiant attitudes have become firmly established.) Parents should also obey these basic rules, as a matter of course.

When children obey family rules, they earn privileges, for example, extra time to watch television or an opportunity to stay up late. Many children like to negotiate, or make lists of, the privileges they want to earn. Earned privileges can be special activities with parents, but children are also motivated by the opportunity to make small purchases, for example, cards (or recently, Webkinz).

Children, when they are not angry or discouraged, want to do well. Almost all children look forward to the opportunity to earn recognition and praise from their parents and teachers. Most young children respond enthusiastically to these simple reward systems—to opportunities to earn stars or stickers, exchanged for privileges—at home and at school.

Parents should always be willing to listen to what their children want—and then let the child know what is possible. With some exceptions (for example, special events that the child learns of at the last minute) negotiations about privileges should take place in advance. Children (especially children who are practiced negotiators) should know that they cannot negotiate all the time and, especially, when a parent has already said, "No." These family rules and limits put into practice a basic principle of emotional maturity that most children come to understand: the child *earns* privileges (and "things") rather than *demanding* them.

The consequences for blatant or egregious violations of rules, like the rules themselves, should also be simple: the child loses a privilege for a relatively brief period of time (for example, an evening of "screen time"). The delineation of reasonable consequences for a child's misbehavior—brief punishments that are easily enforced—may be as important for parents as for children. Managing a child's defiance requires patience and is difficult for all parents. When consequences for the child's violations of rules have been clearly spelled out, parents are more often able to respond calmly (but still firmly), with less anger and retaliation, in these difficult moments. Parents should not have to think up consequences on the spot, or when they are angry, or at their wit's end.

There are many analogies, especially from sports, that children almost universally understand. I remind both parents and children, for example, that a baseball player is allowed (with some restrictions) to argue with an umpire. If he uses profanity, however, or if he continues to argue after the umpire has given him a warning, he is "out of the game" (and, it is instructive to add, a player who touches an umpire during an argument is automatically suspended for three games). Every sport has a similar system of rules—and penalties for infractions—that are well-known to children. And children also generally know (again, until feelings of grievance and defiant attitudes have become habitual) when their behavior is "over the line."

Children understand these rules and *almost always make some initial effort to comply.* This is an essential point: if parents fail to recognize the child's efforts at compliance, or consider them half-hearted or "not enough," the plan will fail. And parents must acknowledge the child's *efforts* as well as his successes ("I could see that you tried really hard to control your temper..."). When parents understand this fundamental principle, they will find many more opportunities to express appreciation and praise. I also encourage parents to offer generous "bonuses" to the child (or, at least, generous expressions of appreciation) for unsolicited pro-social behavior, for example, helping a younger child feel better.

In my experience, when these simple behavioral systems "don't work," other, more serious, family problems have interfered. Parents may consider the plan onerous and therefore fail to follow through. Or parents find it difficult to express frequent appreciation and praise, or they are unable to agree, or an atmosphere of criticism continues unabated. These failures, therefore, are diagnostic, and reveal underlying difficulties that need to be addressed. *We should not be surprised by these difficulties.* Having come to understand the character and philosophy of the parents and the demands they face, both individually and as a couple, we should anticipate and talk with parents, in advance, about possible obstacles and pitfalls in the implementation of any behavioral plan. There is no "right" way of setting limits for children. We need to help parents find a way that works for them.

"They won't stop fighting." Phelan (1995) has presented a technique for managing moments of noncompliance that allows parents to respond to their children's defiant behavior in a calm but still authoritative manner—without yelling and with less arguing—he calls, "1-2-3 Magic." Phelan is right. This method, if not magic, is remarkably effective and helpful to many beleaguered parents—especially, in helping parents respond to fighting among siblings or when children ignore parents' requests. At these moments, parents simply say, "If you don't stop fighting by the time I count to three, you will not be able to... (watch a favorite television program or play a video game)." If used in appropriate contexts, children quickly respond and parents rarely reach the count of three.

In recommending this technique for use in circumscribed problematic situations, I should note that Phelan's approach to parent guidance is, in many respects, antithetical to my own. Although Phelan recognizes the importance of "shared fun" and "active listening," he believes that, in promoting healthy parent-child relationships, effective discipline comes first. (Phelan includes a chapter on active listening at the end, rather than at the beginning, of his book.) In my opinion, listening comes first and discipline is second. Counting to three is an adjunct, certainly not the essence, of good parenting and "The Magic of Encouragement" (Marston, 1990) is far more important than the Magic of 1-2-3.

Tantrums

Tantrums, at any age, are expressions of protest; often, they are expressions of impotent rage. Frequent or prolonged tantrums are a prototype of failed emotional resilience and exhibit all the characteristics of pathological emotional states. In the moment of a tantrum, the child's emotion remains urgent ("I have to have this now") and inflexible (no alternative is acceptable). His thinking is likely to be all-or-nothing and pessimistic ("I *never* get what I want") and he feels a sense of grievance and unfairness.

All children can be expected to vigorously protest—to cry or even to hit—when they are frustrated and disappointed. The extent to which a child (or an adult) is able to respond to common frustrations and disappointments without having a tantrum—to be reasonable in his demands—may serve as a rough measure his emotional maturity. (And a parent's ability to respond to the child's tantrum without "having a tantrum back" may be a measure of a parent's emotional maturity.) In an important sense, all of the recommendations offered in this book—therapeutic strategies that promote the child's increasing ability to tolerate emotional distress, to know that frustrations and disappointments are temporary and therefore bearable, and to take into account the needs of others—are solutions to the problem of a child's tantrums.

Tantrums may also be "manipulative" or coercive. The child may have learned that his tantrums "work"—that if he protests loudly and long enough, his parents will eventually give in, as in the classical coercion model. In these cases, the child has developed a *demand mode* of coping with emotional distress. In my experience, however, coercive tantrums almost always occur in the context of other significant problems in family relationships, for example, lack of positive engagement and supportive listening, severe marital conflict, or persistent criticism.

Frequent tantrums are symptomatic of a child's failure to develop an age-appropriate capacity to tolerate anxiety, frustration, and disappointment and can only be solved *proactively*. All of the elements of proactive problem-solving—appreciation ("validation") of the child's feelings and concerns and the concerns of parents, identifying the likely triggers for a child's tantrums, engaging the child in finding a solution, and establishing reasonable limits on the child's expressions of frustration and disappointment—are necessary components of a plan to reduce the frequency of a child's tantrums. Parents need to help the child learn that disappointments are disappointments, not injustices, and that there will be a "next time" (see Julia, Chapter 2 and Peter, Chapter 10).

Still, parents need to know what to do if a child "freaks out" when a parent says, "No." Almost universally, parents ask, "What punishment should I impose when my child throws the remote control, or screams and speaks abusively when I say, 'No?' " I suggest to parents the following simple rule: if the child has been destructive, whether to objects (if he has broken a toy) or to others (if he has said hurtful things) he must make restitution (for example, apologize) in some form.

Once a tantrum has started, however, there is only patience, calmness, and a firm insistence on behavior that is not destructive or hurtful to others.

Parents should express a willingness to listen to the child's complaint, but only "when you speak to me calmly." I may be among a minority of clinicians in making the following recommendation: if the child calms down and speaks reasonably (not abusively) and if he is able to present a legitimate sense of urgency, parents should, on some occasions, give in to the child's request. I make this recommendation not only because the child has now made a *request* and not a *demand*, but also because allowing the child to feel heard in this way may support his subsequent engagement with us in finding proactive solutions and outweigh the possible risk of reinforcing coercive tactics.

Homework

"Battles" over homework, in my experience,[3] are the most common source of parent-child conflict in middle class, suburban families. In some communities, the amount of time students are expected to spend doing homework far exceeds national recommendations (Cooper, 2001). Many parents accept this conflict with their children as yet another unavoidable consequence of responsible parenting. It is, at best, uncertain, however, whether these battles result in improved learning or performance in school. Even then, the child may (perhaps) eventually be admitted to a prestigious college, but he is now irritable and secretive, or no longer speaks to his parents. Often, battles over homework result in vicious cycles of nagging and avoidance or refusal, with no improvement in the child's school performance and certainly no progress toward what should be our ultimate goal—helping the child develop age-appropriate discipline and independence with respect to schoolwork.

The solution to the problem of homework *always* begins with an accurate diagnosis and a recognition of the demands placed on the child (again, in many cases, we make unreasonable demands). It is worth reiterating: *every* child whose parents or teachers report ongoing resistance to completing schoolwork or homework; *every* child whose performance in school is below expectations based on his parents' or teachers' intuitive assessment of his intellectual potential; and *every* child who, over an extended period of time, complains that he "hates school" or "hates reading," should be evaluated for the presence of an attention or learning disorder *even when other possible pathogenic processes (for example, marital conflict, divorce, or medical illness) are also present.*

These children are not "lazy." The child may be frustrated, discouraged, distracted, anxious, or angry—but this is not laziness. We need to help parents take a step back and reconsider the problem of the child's "motivation." What enables a child to put forth sustained effort on difficult or frustrating tasks—and this is true for all of us, children no less than adults—is the anticipation of future success. Fear of consequences (for example, a bad grade or the disapproval of parents and teachers) may motivate some children to complete their work in the short term, but cannot sustain the child's motivation and effort in the long run. The child's effort eventually fades. Increasingly, he is willing to risk disapproval (or trade certain disapproval) for the short-term relief of anxiety and frustration, and he then develops ways of evading his anxiety with a façade of indifference or "not caring."

Many children who struggle with homework have difficulty getting started. The assigned task—whether because of the demand for sustained attention or, often, for written output—seems overwhelming to the child, as if we were asked to read *War and Peace* in one evening and report on it the following day. The child's refusal or procrastination is an expression of frustration and discouragement, and then protest.

Homework—like any constructive activity—involves moments of anxiety and frustration. Children who have developed a greater capacity to tolerate these unpleasant feelings—children who believe that this work, however onerous, is temporary and therefore bearable and, especially, children who believe that their work will result in some success and recognition of their success—will more effectively cope with this (or any) difficult task.

Still, like many other unpleasant tasks, homework has to be done. If parents begin with at least some understanding of the child's frustration or discouragement, they will be better able to put in place a structure that helps the child learn to work through his frustration—to develop increments of frustration tolerance and self-discipline.

I offer families who struggle with this problem a homework plan. I suggest that parents set aside a specified and limited time for homework—to establish, early in the evening, a homework hour. During this time, all electronics are turned off—for the entire family. Work is done in a communal place, at the kitchen or dining room table. (Contrary to older conventional wisdom, most elementary school children are able to work much more effectively in a common area, with an adult and even other children present, than in the "quiet" of their rooms.) Parents may do their own "homework," but they are present and continually available to help, and to answer children's questions. The goal is to create, to the extent possible, a library atmosphere in the home, again, for a specified—and limited—period of time. Ideally, therefore, parents should not make or receive telephone calls during this hour. And when homework is done, there is time for play.[4]

Most families have found these suggestions helpful, especially for elementary school children.[5] Establishing a homework hour allows parents to move away from threats ("If you don't...") to opportunities ("When you have finished...we'll have a chance to..."). Of course, for many hurried or disorganized families, there are complications and potential glitches in implementing any homework plan. But parents should not use the complications of scheduling or other competing demands as a reason not to establish a reasonable homework routine.

Sleep

Many parents express concern that their child has difficulty falling asleep at night. The child wants a parent (or a sibling) to stay with him until he falls asleep; if the parent leaves, he finds reasons to repeatedly call for his parent or come out of his room. He may (or may not) report specific anxieties, for example, a fear of monsters or intruders; often, he says that he "just feels scared." Over time, his parents are exhausted.

As we get to know the child, we may suspect different causes for his difficulty going to sleep. Many children are anxious about going to school the following day. These children often present a "Sunday night syndrome" (not unlike many adults who are unable to fall asleep in anticipation of job-related stress) and they may fall asleep easily on weekend nights. Other children have become angry; their difficulty falling asleep reflects a conscious or unconscious preoccupation with angry thoughts. Or the child's difficulty falling asleep may have begun during a period of separation from his parents. For perhaps the majority of children with sleep difficulties, however, we may find no "reason" for their sleep disturbance; instead, we may reasonably suspect a biologically-based anxiety sensitivity—an increased fear of separation or fear of the dark that is instinctive in all children. And even when we have developed a plausible explanation of the child's fear, this understanding often does not help us solve the problem.[6]

In helping a child fall asleep, parents should begin with all the common elements a soothing bedtime routine: a regular bedtime, transitional objects, reading or telling a story, and time for the child to talk about any of his concerns—problems of the day or, especially, worries about the following day. Many children also derive comfort from being able to help their dolls or stuffed animals go to sleep and feel better. Despite these solacing rituals, however, many children remain afraid and ask their parents to stay with them until they fall asleep. Some parents have attempted to solve this problem with rewards (for remaining in the room) or punishments (for leaving the room); in my experience, these measures are rarely effective.

I recommend to parents a plan that helps almost all children learn to overcome nighttime separation anxiety. After the regular bedtime rituals, parents explain to the child that they will leave the room, but then come back, to check on the child, at regular intervals. Depending on the age of the child and the intensity of the child's fear, parents should return to the child's room every 5 or 10 minutes, and then at increasing intervals, over the course of the next few weeks. In this way, *the child learns, in manageable increments, to tolerate being alone, because he anticipates the parent's return.*[7] Almost all children cooperate with this plan (because the child, although he is afraid, wants to overcome his fear). Some parents object to the initial increase in time and effort involved in this intervention. Returning to check on the child, however, requires less time and effort than responding—with increasing irritation—to the child's requests. Of course, the parent must return as promised, before the child calls for her or leaves his room; if the parent waits until the child calls, the child has learned the wrong lesson. Although reward systems for helping a child overcome nighttime fears are usually unsuccessful, a parent can add rewards as an additional incentive. The problem of children who wake up in the middle of the night is more difficult to solve and takes more time; however, when the going-to-sleep problem is resolved, the middle-of-the-night problem is less burdensome and, most often, gradually fades.

The 15-Minute Rule

Schwartz (1996) has presented an empirically-validated therapeutic intervention for adult patients with OCD (adapted as a self-help program) that is extremely valuable in solving many childhood problems. The Schwartz treatment model is based on a simple, but critical, observation: that patients—including children—are generally able to stop performing a compulsive behavior (for example, compulsive hand washing) for short periods of time, *if they know that they will be able to resume the behavior at some later time.* This simple observation then leads to a highly effective therapeutic technique. In the case of compulsive hand washing, the patient is told to stop washing for 15 minutes. During this time, he performs some pleasurable behavior as a distraction and is then free to resume the compulsive behavior at the agreed upon time. Intervals between compulsive behaviors are then lengthened, in manageable increments. The patient learns, in this way, to tolerate longer periods of time without carrying out a ritual or compulsion, and now has much longer periods of compulsion-free time. In addition, what was formerly a compulsive behavior has now been transformed, at least to some degree, into a *voluntary* behavior, that is, the patient now decides whether or not he needs to resume washing.

This step in the Schwartz self-help program—the 15-minute rule—can be adapted for many problematic behaviors of childhood. This technique is helpful to parents in managing any behavior a child is unable or unwilling to stop or any anxiety a child is unable to tolerate, including worries that are not true obsessions or behaviors that are not true compulsions, for example, repeated requests of any kind. The child is able to inhibit his behavior—or postpone his demands—because he knows the discussion will continue at a later time. A parent can say to a child, for example, who repeatedly asks "Will you buy me..." or "I want..." or makes other insistent demands, that the parent will no longer talk about this problem now, but will talk again at a specified time. The child, although frustrated, learns to tolerate a small increment of anxiety or frustration—because his concerns have not been dismissed and will be addressed later—and parents are less likely to become angry and threaten punishment.

Television and Electronic Games

The fascination of children and adolescents with television and electronic games, especially games and programs with violent content, is of increasing concern to many contemporary families. We are often told, "All he wants to do is play Game Boy or video games." Many adolescents—players and former players—openly acknowledge the addictive quality of these games (and will tell us, when we ask, which games are more, or less, addictive). Singer and Singer (2005), based on a review of several decades of research, including longitudinal studies, have raised significant concern about the deleterious effects on children of frequent watching of violent television programs and playing violent video games. Singer and Singer report that, contrary to their initial expectations (and my own), strong evidence now exists for a causal, not merely correlational, relationship between television and video game violence and subsequent aggressive behavior in children and adolescents.[8]

The problem of how, and to what extent, parents should limit the child's watching television or playing video games is difficult, and we need to admit our uncertainty. Most often (although perhaps not always) a child's "addiction" to electronics is symptomatic of some other underlying problem, for example, discouragement or social isolation, or, in some cases, a family atmosphere of frequent conflict or ineffective discipline (families, for example, in which children ignore parents' stated rules and parents then admonish their children and threaten punishments, but do not follow through). Excessive screen time is also a frequent problem in families where both parents work extended hours and children are supervised by caregivers who lack the authority to enforce rules. Despite our uncertainty, however, parents need a plan.

Many families have found the following guidelines helpful:

(1) Substitute interactive play for electronic play. Most children, despite some perfunctory protests, still prefer interactive play with a parent to television and video games, with all the benefits discussed above.

(2) Set aside a specified time for video games and a specified time during which television and electronics are turned off.

(3) I have also, at times, made what may appear to be a more radical proposal: parents should play electronic games with the child. Parents can watch the child play and ask him to teach them the game. This recommendation is an extension of the principle that parents should express interest in the child's interests. Almost all children want their parents to watch them play these games, so that they can show off their skill. The results of this informal experiment have been encouraging. Parents usually report, as predicted, that the child is more willing, at a later time, to engage with them in non-electronic activities.

(4) Game time can be earned—as a reward for compliance with basic responsibilities.

At School: A Book of Positives

Teachers also ask for our help. Many schools have now implemented reward-based behavior management programs for children with problems of impulse control and affect regulation or social skills education for students, to help children respond appropriately in problematic peer interactions. School-based programs have also been developed for the development of improved executive functions and behavior regulation (Webster-Stratton, 2003; Greenberg, 2006).

For individual teachers, especially in schools where formal programs have not yet been established, the following recommendations are often helpful. Our advice to teachers will vary, of course, depending on our understanding of each individual child. We begin, as always, by helping teachers recognize the sources of a child's frustration and discouragement, and then to provide acknowledgement and praise for each increment in the child's ability to "handle" his emotions and every advance in the child's pro-social behavior. The "language of becoming" that is essential for parents and therapists is important for teachers as well.

I often recommend that parents and teachers create for the child a "Book of Positives." The child's teacher is asked to write at least one positive comment about the child each day—a statement of appreciation, for example, of the child's effort at self control or his helpfulness to a classmate or a younger child. And I encourage teachers to create opportunities for the child to earn recognition, especially for pro-social behaviors. The child takes his book home each night, and his parents add a positive comment. This simple technique is not a cure for severe problems of behavior or affect dysregulation, but has reparative value for many young children and often begins to interrupt vicious cycles of criticism and defiance that commonly occur in school as well as at home.

Notes

1. Recent research has raised important questions about the kind of praise we should offer children, especially, the negative effects of praising children's *abiities*, rather than their *effort.* Dweck (2002; 2004; Mueller and Dweck, 1998), in a series of important studies, has distinguished two types of beliefs that children (and adults) hold about the nature of our abilities. Children who are "entity" theorists regard abilities, including intelligence, as stable internal traits; "incremental" theorists, in contrast, believe that abilities are malleable and can improve with effort. Dweck's research demonstrates that children who hold an incremental theory of ability show more optimism and persistence than entity theorists when they are faced with setbacks. And, in a study that has special relevance, Mueller and Dweck (1998) report that children who were praised for their *intelligence,* rather than their *effort*, showed less persistence and less task enjoyment when they were presented with challenging problems at a later time.

Kohn (1993) has argued strongly against the use of rewards, including praise, in the socialization of children. He warns that rewards have, at best, short-term effectiveness and that frequent praise undermines the child's intrinsic motivations and confidence in his independent judgment.

In the popular press, these ideas have been widely publicized, often under the misleading title, "the over-praised child." Kohn's arguments have some merit, and the question of what kind of praise may be either beneficial or harmful to children deserves careful study. It should be clear that I am recommending frequent praise (and expressions of appreciation) for the child's effort, not praise for innate ability, and I certainly do not recommend praise that is unrealistic or insincere. I am concerned, however, about the popularization of the concept of an "over-praised" child. Although this syndrome may exist (and may even be prevalent), in several decades of clinical practice, I have met many discouraged, angry, and unhappy children and the culprit is not praise, but criticism. Most of these children were over-criticized; very few were "over-praised."

2. For some families, there is a third category of rules—rules necessary to promote values that are particularly important to a given family (for example, restrictions on watching television or playing violent video games or attendance at religious observances).
3. But not only in my experience. A decade ago, Piscataway, NJ, because of concerns that homework demands were having a destructive effect on family life, limited the amount of homework teachers could assign to a maximum of 30 minutes per day for elementary school students and 2 hours for high school students. The long-term success of this—in my opinion, very reasonable—experiment is, of course, unknown and difficult to evaluate. Media reports at the time, however, indicated that the Piscataway plan was greeted approvingly by a large majority of parents in the community.

   Cooper (2001), based on a comprehensive review of research on homework, recommends that school districts adopt a "10-minute rule"—students and parents "should expect all homework assignments together to last as long as 10 minutes multiplied by the student's grade level" (or perhaps 15 minutes if required reading time is included). Cooper suggests that beyond 15 minutes per grade, "the costs of homework will begin to outweigh the benefits (p. 65)."
4. When there are frequent battles and bad feelings over how well the child has done his homework, whether he has made a good-enough effort, I have, at times, made a radical suggestion: parents do not have to check to see if the child's homework is correct; the child's teacher will do this the following day.
5. The problem of procrastination among middle school and high school students is more difficult. Despite my offer to many teenagers to collaborate on a bestselling book, "The Cure for Procrastination," the book remains unwritten and the problem is often intractable.
6. On some occasions, we may be able, through an analysis of the child's fantasies or dreams, to develop an understanding of the child's fear that we can then communicate to the child and that resolves his sleep disturbance. Shapiro (1983) has reported a case in which a young child's nighttime anxiety was the result of a confusion of sleep and death. But these cases constitute a small minority.

7. In behaviorist approaches to helping children fall asleep—without calling for their parents or leaving their room—this element of a bedtime plan (similar in implementation, although based on a different understanding of the child's experience than the approach I am recommending) is called by the misleading name, "graduated extinction" (Rabian and Bottjer, 2008).
8. Singer and Singer note that, in many of the studies reviewed, "the outcome measures were by no means trivial" (2005, p. 96) and included violent behavior in adolescence and adulthood. The authors also cite additional evidence for the relationship of television violence and aggressive behavior based on intervention research. Intervention studies in schools have demonstrated that educational programs designed to promote "critical viewing" of television resulted in both decreased viewing of violent shows and decreased aggressive behavior.

   Singer and Singer suggest that excessive involvement in these activities results, especially, in "a narrowing of one's imaginative range" (p. 102) and "a repetitive over-learning of schemas or scripts involving aggression" (p. 104). They conclude that the results of this research "are of sufficient magnitude to be considered public health problems of almost the same order as the research on smoking and lung cancer, lead exposure and intellectual deficits, or condom use in reducing HIV transmission" (pp. 101–102).

Epilogue

The project of child psychotherapy is now a century old. In the early years of the twentieth century, impulsive or hyperactive children were thought to suffer from "a defect in moral control" (Still, cited in Barkley, 1990) and Freud (1909) remarked that the common phobias of children, "decidedly inconvenient" for caregivers, were often "shouted down in the nursery" (p. 142). Now, of course, we regard children's emotional and behavioral problems with both greater compassion and scientific understanding. All of the major traditions of psychotherapy—humanistic, psychodynamic, cognitive, and behavioral—have developed concepts and methods that have advanced our ability to offer help to troubled children and families.

Each of these traditions retains a distinctive focus and offers a distinctive contribution to our understanding of child development and the process of therapeutic change. Humanistic theory reminds us of the importance of empathy and acceptance; psychodynamic theory teaches us about the child's conflicts, her motives for resistance, and her ongoing need for experiences of affirmation and idealization; cognitive theory attempts to diminish the power of the child's pathogenic beliefs and improve her problem-solving skills; and behavioral theory has identified pathogenic family processes and demonstrated the importance of frequent positive reinforcement in strengthening pro-social behaviors in defiant children.

Recent developmental research has also made significant contributions to our understanding of optimal and pathological development in childhood. We now have strong evidence for the importance of a secure attachment relationship and of interactive repair processes in promoting the child's positive expectations—expectations that are vital to emotional health. Clinical, developmental, and neuroscience studies have demonstrated the importance of interactive play, and of emotional communication and emotional reciprocity, in helping children establish successful peer relationships and a "moral self."

In this book, I have offered my own clinical understanding—an emotion-based perspective that highlights the pathogenic pathways of demoralization and defiance and the critical role of reparative mechanisms in sustaining the child's positive emotions. From this perspective, the essence of our therapeutic task is to promote emotional resilience: to arrest the spread of malignant events in the mind of the child, strengthen the child's expectation of affirming responsiveness, and restore more optimistic beliefs about her future.

* * *

Therapists of different schools are, at times, dismissive of the methods used by alternative approaches. But they should not be. The diversity of childhood problems—and the complexity of each individual case—require a diversity of therapeutic techniques. Strict adherence to any theoretical model limits the range of children we will be able to help. As our therapeutic strategies continue to be refined, differences between schools have become less prominent. A consensus has emerged: improved emotion regulation (or, as I prefer, emotional resilience) is now regarded as a critical achievement in normal development and a goal of most therapeutic interventions for troubled children.

I hope that the ideas presented in this book will contribute, in some measure, to a dialogue among therapists of different schools and an integration of competing therapeutic models. The clinical problems I have discussed—how to engage a child in therapy, how to mitigate a child's (and family's) resistance, and how to promote a child's pro-social development—are problems faced, at some time, by every child therapist. Behavioral and cognitive-behavioral therapists will benefit, I believe, from increased understanding of the child's emotions (for example, the emotions of interest, shame, and pride) and from a greater appreciation of therapeutic processes—especially, empathy—that directly influence the child's emotional experience. And I would encourage humanistic and psychodynamic child therapists to make greater use of proven cognitive-behavioral techniques—in helping children with symptoms of anxiety and depression and in resolving common problems of daily living that are the bane of so many modern families.

Kendall (2006) advises that we should be realistic in our therapeutic aspirations. He correctly notes that successful child therapy does not cure an illness but, instead, helps to alter a pathological trajectory. (Kendall reminds us that even Michael Jordan was able to make less than half of the shots he took.) There is some wisdom in these observations. Our therapeutic success will always be subject to limitations. We will be consulted by children and families where malignant processes have spread extensively—where the child's demoralization and defiant attitudes have become deeply ingrained and the child's or family's resistances are tenacious. In other cases, our success will be constrained by biological factors that are strongly present and difficult to mitigate; or by our own, inevitable, personal failures.

I would offer, however, a more optimistic assessment. If we avail ourselves of a comprehensive understanding of a child's emotional development—and a range of strategies to help both children and parents—we will be able, far more often than not, to set in motion a therapeutic process and make substantial progress toward the goals we hope to achieve: to restore affirming responsiveness between parents and their children, ameliorate the child's demoralization and defiant attitudes, and promote the child's initiative and pro-social development—changes that will be of lasting benefit in the lives of children and their parents.

References

Abraham, K. (1921/1927). Contributions to the Theory of the Anal Character. In *Selected Papers on Psychoanalysis.* London: Karnac Books, 370–392.

Achenbach, T. M., Howell, C. T., Quay, H. C., and Conners, C. K. (1991). National Survey of Problems and Competencies Among 4- to 16-Year-Olds: Parents' Reports for Normative and Clinical Samples. *Monographs of the Society for Research in Child Development, 56* (Serial No. 225).

Adams-Silvan, A. and Silvan, M. (1988). On Transitionality and Defects in Empathic Capacity: A Clinical and Theoretical Study. In P. Horton, H. Gewirtz, and K. J. Kreutter (Eds.) *The Solace Paradigm: An Eclectic Search for Psychological Immunity.* Madison, CT: International Universities Press, 341–379.

Alloy, L., Abramson, L., Tashman, N., Berreddi, D., Hogan, M., Whitehouse, W., Crossfield, A., and Morocco, A. (2001). Developmental Origins of Cognitive Vulnerability to Depression: Parenting, Cognitive, and Inferential Feedback Styles of Parents of Individuals at High and Low Cognitive Risk for Depression. *Cognitive Therapy and Research,* 25(4), 397–423.

Altman, N., Briggs, R., Frankel, J., Gensler, D., and Pantone, P. (2002). *Relational Child Psychotherapy.* New York: Other Press.

Axline, V. (1947). *Play Therapy.* New York: Balantine Books.

Bach, S. (1994). Being Heard: Attunement and the Growth of Psychic Structure. In *The Language of Perversion and the Language of Love.* Northvale, NJ: Jason Aronson, 141–162.

Barish, K. (2004). The Child Therapist's Generative Use of Self. *Journal of Infant, Child, and Adolescent Psychotherapy,* Vol. 3, No. 2, 270–282.

Barkley, R. (1990). *Attention-Deficit Hyperactivity Disorder: A Handbook for Diagnosis and Treatment.* New York: Guilford Press.

Barkley, R. (1997a). *ADHD and the Nature of Self-Control.* New York: Guilford Press.

Barkley, R. (1997b). *Defiant Children (2nd Ed.): A Clinician's Manual For Assessment and Parent Training.* New York: Guilford Press.

Baron-Cohen, S. (2003). *The Essential Difference.* New York: Basic Books.

Barrett, K. C. (1995). A Functionalist Approach to Shame and Guilt. In J. P. Tangney and K. W. Fischer (Eds.) *Self-Conscious Emotions: The Psychology of Shame, Guilt, Embarrassment, and Pride.* New York: Guilford Press.

Barrett, K. C. (1998). A Functionalist Perspective to the Development of Emotions. In M. F. Mascolo and S. Griffin (Eds.) *What Develops in Emotional Development?* New York: Plenum Press, 109–158.

Barrett, K. C. and Campos, J. J. (1987). Perspectives on Emotional Development: II. A Functionalist Approach to Emotions. In J. Osofsky (Ed.) *Handbook of Infant Development*, 2nd Ed. New York: Wiley, 555–578.

Barr-Zisowitz, C. (2000). "Sadness"—Is There Such a Thing? In M. Lewis and J. M. Haviland-Jones (Eds.) *Handbook of Emotions*, 2nd Ed. New York: Guilford Press, 607–622.

Basch, M. F. (1982). Dynamic Psychotherapy and Its Frustrations. In P. L. Wachtel (Ed.) *Resistance: Psychodynamic and Behavioral Approaches*. New York: Plenum Press, 3–24.

Bellinson, J. (2002). *Children's Use of Board Games in Psychotherapy*. Northvale, NJ: Jason Aronson.

Benjamin, J. (1988). *The Bonds of Love*. New York: Pantheon Books.

Benjamin J. (1995). *Like Subjects, Love Objects: Essays on Recognition and Sexual Difference*. New Haven, CT: Yale University Press.

Beren, P. (1998). Narcissism and Oedipal Development. In P. Beren (Ed.) *Narcissistic Disorders in Children and Adolescents: Diagnosis and Treatment*. Northvale, NJ: Jason Aronson, 67–83.

Biederman, J., Rosenbaum, J. F., Bolduc-Murphy, E. A., Faraone, S., Chaloff, J., Hirschfeld, D. R., and Kagan, J. (1993). Behavioral Inhibition as a Temperamental Risk Factor for Anxiety Disorders. *Child and Adolescent Psychiatric Clinics of North America*, Vol. 2, 667–684.

Blatt, S. and Behrends, R. S. (1987). Internalization, Separation-Individuation, and the Nature of Therapeutic Action. *International Journal of Psychoanalysis*, Vol. 68, 279–297.

Bleiberg, E., Fonagy, P., and Target, M. (1997). Child Psychoanalysis: Critical Overview and a Proposed Re-consideration. *Child and Adolescent Psychiatric Clinics of North America*, Vol. 6, No. 1, 1–38.

Bloom, P. (2004). *Descartes' Baby: How the Science of Child Development Explains What Makes Us Human*. New York: Basic Books.

Bonanno, G. A. and Mayne, T. J. (2001). The Future of Emotion Research. In T. Mayne and G. Bonanno (Eds.) *Emotions: Current Issues and Future Directions*. New York: Guilford Press, 398–410.

Bowlby, J. (1980). *Loss: Sadness and Depression*. New York: Basic Books.

Bradley, S. (2000). *Affect Regulation and the Development of Psychopathology*. New York: Guilford Press.

Bromfield, R. (2007). *Doing Child and Adolescent Psychotherapy: Adapting Psychodynamic Treatment to Contemporary Practice* (2nd Ed.). Hoboken, NJ: John Wiley and Sons.

Brooks, D. (2007). Goodbye, George and John. *New York Times*, August 8, 2007.

Brooks, R. (2006). The Power of Parenting. In R. Brooks and S. Goldstein (Eds.) *Handbook of Resilience in Children*. New York: Springer, 297–314.

Capobianco, J. and Farber, B. A. (2005). Therapist Self-Disclosure to Child Patients. *American Journal of Psychotherapy*, Vol. 59, No. 3, 199–212.

Cavell, T. (2000). *Working with Parents of Aggressive Children: A Practitioner's Guide*. Washington, DC: American Psychological Association.

Chassequet-Smirgel, J. (1985). *The Ego-Ideal: A Psychoanalytic Essay on the Malady of the Ideal*. London: Free Association Books.

Chethik, M. (2000). *Techniques of Child Therapy: Psychodynamic Strategies*, 2nd Ed. New York: Guilford Press.

Chorpita, B. (2001). Control and the Development of Negative Emotions. In M. W. Vasey and M. R. Dadds (Eds.) *The Developmental Psychopathology of Anxiety.* New York: Oxford University Press, 112–142.

Chused, J. (2004). *The Evolving Nature of Transference in Child Analysis.* Paper presented at Symposium 2004: Contemporary Psychoanalytic Perspectives on Transference. New York, February 2004.

Cicchetti, D. and Cohen, D. (Eds.) (2006). *Developmental Psychopathology*, 2nd Ed. Hoboken, NJ: John Wiley and Sons.

Clark, L. A. and Watson, D. (1994). Distinguishing Functional from Dysfunctional Affective Responses. In P. Ekman and R. J. Davidson (Eds.) *The Nature of Emotion: Fundamental Questions.* New York: Oxford University Press, 131–136.

Cohen, P. and Solnit, A. (1993). Play and Therapeutic Action. *Psychoanalytic Study of the Child*, Vol. 48, 49–63.

Cole, P. M. and Zahn-Waxler, C. (1992). Emotional Dysregulation in Disruptive Behavior Disorders. In D. Cicchetti and S. L. Toth (Eds.) *Rochester Symposium on Developmental Psychopathology: Developmental Perspectives on Depression*, Vol. 4. Rochester, NY: University of Rochester Press, 173–209.

Coleridge, S. T. (1952). The Rime of the Ancient Mariner. In O. Williams (Ed.) *Immortal Poems of the English Language.* New York: Washington Square Press.

Conner, T. and Barrett, L. F. (2005). Implicit Self-Attitudes Predict Spontaneous Affect in Daily Life. *Emotion*, Vol. 4, No. 5, 476–488.

Cooper, H. (2001). *The Battle Over Homework* (2nd Ed.). Thousand Oaks, CA: Corwin Press.

Cummings, E. M. and Davies, P. (1995). The Impact of Parents on Their Children: An Emotional Security Perspective. *Annals of Child Development*, Vol. 10, 167–208.

Cummings, E. M. and Davies, P. (1996). Emotional Security as a Regulatory Process in Normal Development and the Development of Psychopathology. *Development and Psychopathology*, Vol. 8, 123–139.

Damasio, A. R. (1994). *Descartes' Error: Emotion, Reason, and the Human Brain.* New York: G. P. Putman.

Davidson, R. J. (1994). On Emotion, Mood, and Related Affective Constructs. In P. Ekman and R. J. Davidson (Eds.) *The Nature of Emotion: Fundamental Questions.* New York: Oxford University Press, 51–55.

Davies, P. and Cummings, E. M. (1995). Children's Emotions as Organizers of Their Reactions to Interadult Anger: A Functionalist Perspective. *Developmental Psychology*, Vol. 31, No. 4, 677–684.

Demos, E. V. (1984). Empathy and Affect: Reflections on Infant Experience. In J. Lichtenberg (Ed.) *Empathy.* Hillsdale, NJ: Analytic Press.

Demos, E. V. (1995). *Exploring Affect: The Selected Writings of Silvan Tomkins.* Cambridge: Cambridge University Press.

DeWaal, F. (2001). *The Ape and the Sushi Master.* New York: Basic Books.

Dix, T. (1991). The Affective Organization of Parenting. *Psychological Bulletin*, Vol. 110, No. 1, 3–25.

Dizdar, M., Rodriquez, H., Jaruga, P., and Birincioglu, M. (2003). Oxidative Stress/DNA Damage and DNA Repair. www.cstl.nist.gov/biotech/DNAtech/WebPageDNAdamage.html. Last accessed: June 4, 2004.

Dodge, K. A., Bates, J. E., and Petit, G. S. (1990). Mechanisms in the Cycle of Violence. *Science,* Vol. 250, 1678–1683.

Drucker, J. (1994). Constructing Metaphors: The Role of Symbolization in the Treatment of Children. In A. Slade and D. P. Wolf (Eds.) *Children at Play.* New York: Oxford University Press, 62–80.

Dumas, J. E. and LaFreniere, P. (1993). Mother-Child Relationships as Sources of Support or Stress: A Comparison of Competent, Average, Aggressive, and Anxious Dyads. *Child Development,* Vol. 64: 1732–1754.

Dunn, J. and Brown, J. (1991). Relationships, Talk about Feelings, and the Development of Affect Regulation in Early Childhood. In J. Garber and K. A. Dodge (Eds.) *The Development of Emotion Regulation and Dysregulation.* Cambridge: Cambridge University Press, 89–108.

Dweck, C. S. (2002). The Development of Ability Conceptions. In J. S. Eccles and A. Wigfield (Eds.) *Development of Achievement Motivation.* San Diego, CA: Academic Press, 57–88.

Dweck, C. S. (2004). The Role of Mental Representation in Social Development. *Merrill-Palmer Quarterly,* Vol. 50, No. 4, October 2004, 428–444.

Eisenberg, N. (2000). Empathy and Sympathy. In M. Lewis and J. M. Haviland-Jones, (Eds.) *Handbook of Emotions,* 2nd Ed. New York: Guilford Press, 677–692.

Elson, M. (Ed.) (1987). *The Kohut Seminars on Self Psychology and Psychotherapy with Adolescents and Young Adults.* New York: W. W. Norton.

Emde, R. (1991). Positive Emotions for Psychoanalytic Theory: Surprises from Infancy Research and New Directions. *Journal of the American Psychoanalytic Association,* Vol. 39, 3–44.

Erikson, E. (1950). *Childhood and Society.* New York: W. W. Norton.

Erikson, E. (1959). *Identity and the Life Cycle.* New York: W. W. Norton.

Feshbach, N. (1989). Empathy Training. In J. Groebel and R. Hinde (Eds.) *Aggression and War: Their Biological and Social Bases.* Cambridge: Cambridge University Press, 101–111.

Fischer, K. W. and Tangney, J. P. (1995). Self-Conscious Emotions and the Affect Revolution: Framework and Overview. In J. P. Tangney and K. W. Fischer (Eds.) *Self-Conscious Emotions: The Psychology of Shame, Guilt, Embarrassment, and Pride.* New York: Guilford Press, 3–22.

Fischer, K. W., Shaver, P. R., and Carnochan, P. (1990). How Emotions Develop and How they Organize Development. *Cognition and Emotion,* Vol. 4, No. 2, 81–12.

Fonagy, P. (2004). Psychodynamic Therapy with Children. In H. Steiner (Ed.) *Handbook of Mental Health Interventions in Children and Adolescents.* San Francisco, CA: Jossey-Bass, 621–658.

Fonagy, P. and Target, M. (1998). Mentalization and the Changing Aims of Child Psychoanalysis. *Psychoanalytic Dialogues,* Vol. 8, No. 1, 87–114.

Fonagy, P., Moran, G., and Target, M. (1993). Aggression and the Psychological Self. *International Journal of Psychoanalysis,* Vol. 74, 471–485.

Fonagy, P., Gergely, G., Jurist, E., and Target, M. (2002*). Affect Regulation, Mentalization, and the Development of the Self.* New York: Other Press.

Fonagy, P., Target, M., Cottrell, D., Phillips, J., and Kurtz, Z. (2002). *What Works for Whom? A Critical Review of Treatments for Children and Adolescents.* New York: Guilford Press.

Forehand, R. and Long, N. (1996). *Parenting the Strong-Willed Child.* Chicago, IL: Contemporary Books.

Forgatch, M. S., Bullock, B. M., and Patterson, G. R. (2004). From Theory to Practice: Increasing Effective Parenting through Role-Play. In H. Steiner (Ed.) *Handbook of Mental Health Interventions in Children and Adolescents*. San Francisco, CA: Jossey-Bass, 782–813.

Frank, J. D. and Frank, J. B. (1961/1991). *Persuasion and Healing,* 3rd Ed. Baltimore, MD: Johns Hopkins University Press.

Frankel, J. B. (1998). The Play's the Thing: How the Essential Processes of Therapy Are Seen Most Clearly in Child Therapy. *Psychoanalytic Dialogues*, Vol. 8, No. 1, 149–182.

Fredrickson, B. (1998). What Good Are Positive Emotions? *Review of General Psychology*, Vol. 2, No. 3, 300–319.

Fredrickson, B. and Branigan, C. (2001). Positive Emotions. In T. Mayne and G. Bonanno (Eds.) *Emotions: Current Issues and Future Directions*. New York: Guilford Press, 123–151.

Freud, A. (1946). *The Psychoanalytical Treatment of Children*. London: Imago.

Freud, A. (1974). A Psychoanalytic View of Developmental Psychopathology. In *The Writings of Anna Freud*, Vol. 8. New York: International Universities Press.

Freud, S. (1909). Analysis of a Phobia in a Five-Year-Old Boy. *Standard Edition*, X: 5–149. London: Hogarth Press.

Freud, S. (1911). Formulations on the Two Principles of Mental Functioning. *Standard Edition,* XI: 218–226. London: Hogarth Press.

Freud, S. (1912). Recommendations to Physicians Practicing Psychoanalysis. *Standard Edition,* XII: 109–120. London: Hogarth Press.

Freud, S. (1914). On The History of the Psychoanalytic Movement. *Standard Edition,* XIV: 7–66. London: Hogarth Press.

Freud, S. (1921). Group Psychology and the Analysis of the Ego. *Standard Edition*, XVIII: 67–143. London: Hogarth Press.

Freud, S. (1926). Inhibitions, Symptoms and Anxiety. *Standard Edition*, XX: 77–178. London: Hogarth Press.

Frijda, N. (1994). Emotions Are Functional, Most of the Time. In P. Ekman and R. J. Davidson (Eds.) *The Nature of Emotion: Fundamental Questions*. New York: Oxford University Press, 112–122.

Frijda, N. (2000). The Psychologist's Point of View. In M. Lewis and J. M. Haviland-Jones (Eds.) *Handbook of Emotions*, 2nd Ed. NY: Guilford Press, 59–74.

Frijda, N. (2007). *The Laws of Emotion*. Mahwah, NJ: Lawrence Erlbaum Associates.

Gaines, R. (1995). The Treatment of Children. In M. Lionells, C. Mann, J. Fiscalini, and D. B. Stern (Eds.) *Handbook of Interpersonal Psychoanalysis*. Hillsdale, NJ: Analytic Press.

Gallese, V. (2001). The "Shared Manifold" Hypothesis: From Mirror Neurons to Empathy. *Journal of Consciousness Studies,* Vol. 8, Nos. 5–7, 33–50.

Gardner, H. (1983). *Frames of Mind*. New York: Basic Books.

Gilbert, P. (2003). Evolution, Social Roles, and the Differences in Shame and Guilt. *Social Research*, Vol. 70, No. 4, 1205–1230.

Gilbert, P. and McGuire, M. T. (1998). Shame, Status, and Social Roles: Psychobiology and Evolution. In P. Gilbert and B. Andrews (Eds.) *Shame: Interpersonal Behavior, Psychopathology, and Culture*. New York: Oxford University Press, 99–125.

Gilligan, J. (2003). Shame, Guilt, and Violence. *Social Research*, Vol. 70, No. 4, 1149–1180.

Ginott, H. (1965). *Between Parent and Child.* New York: Three Rivers Press.
Goleman, D. (2003). *Destructive Emotions.* New York: Random House.
Gotthold, J. (1996). It's as Easy as Child's Play: Play, A Self Psychological Understanding. *Psychoanalysis and Psychotherapy*, Vol. 13, No. 1, 19–26.
Gottman, J. M. (1994). *What Predicts Divorce? The Relationship between Marital Processes and Marital Outcomes.* Hillsdale, NJ: Lawrence Erlbaum Associates.
Gottman, J. M. (1997). *The Heart of Parenting.* New York: Simon & Schuster.
Gottman, J. M., Katz, L., and Hooven, C. (1997). *Meta-Emotion: How Families Communicate Emotionally.* Mahwah, NJ: Lawrence Erlbaum Associates.
Granic, I. and Patterson, G. R. (2006). Toward a Comprehensive Model of Antisocial Development: A Dynamic Systems Approach. *Psychological Review*, Vol. 113, No. 1, 101–131.
Greenberg, M. (2006). Promoting Resilience in Children and Youth: Preventive Interventions and Their Interface with Neuroscience. In M. Lester, A. Masten, and B. McEwan (Eds.) *Resilience in Children. Annals of the New York Academy of Sciences*, Vol. 1094, 139–150.
Greene, R. W. (1998). *The Explosive Child.* New York: HarperCollins.
Greene, R. W. and Ablon, J. S. (2006). *Treating Explosive Kids.* New York: Guilford Press.
Greenspan, S. (1993). *Playground Politics.* Reading, MA: Addison-Wesley.
Greenspan, S. (1995). *The Challenging Child.* Reading, MA: Addison-Wesley.
Greenspan, S. (1997). *The Growth of the Mind and the Endangered Origins of Intelligence.* Reading, MA: Addison-Wesley.
Greenspan, S. and Wieder, S. (1997). Developmental Patterns and Outcomes in Infants and Children with Disorders of Relating and Communicating: A Chart Review of 200 Cases of Children with Autistic Spectrum Diagnoses. *Journal of Developmental and Learning Disorders*, Vol. 1, 87–143.
Greenspan, S. and Wieder, S. (1998). *The Child with Special Needs.* Reading, MA: Perseus Books.
Griffin, S. and Mascolo, M. F. (1998). On the Nature, Development, and Function of Emotions. In M. F. Mascolo and S. Griffin (Eds.) *What Develops in Emotional Development?* New York: Plenum Press, 3–27.
Gross, J. J. and Thompson, R. A. (2007). Emotion Regulation: Conceptual Foundations. In J. J. Gross (Ed.) *Handbook of Emotion Regulation.* New York: Guilford Press.
Halpern, J. (2001). *From Detached Concern to Empathy: Humanizing Medical Practice.* New York: Oxford University Press.
Harter, S. (1988). Developmental and Dynamic Changes in the Nature of the Self-Concept: Implications for Child Psychotherapy. In S. Shirk (Ed.) *Cognitive Development and Child Psychotherapy.* New York: Plenum Press.
Hooven, C., Gottman, J. M., and Katz, L. (1995). Parental Meta-Emotion Structure Predicts Family and Child Outcomes. *Cognition and Emotion,* Vol. 9, No. 2/3, 229–264.
Horton, P. and Gerwitz, H. (1988). Acquisition and Termination of First Solacing Objects in Males, Females and in a Clinic and Non-Clinic Population: Implications for Psychological Immunity. In P. Horton, H. Gewirtz, and K. J. Kreutter (Eds.) *The Solace Paradigm: An Eclectic Search for Psychological Immunity.* Madison, CT: International Universities Press, 159–183.
Izard, C. (1991). *The Psychology of Emotions.* New York: Plenum Press.

Izard, C. E. and Ackerman, B. P. (2000). Motivational, Organizational, and Regulatory Functions of Discrete Emotions, In M. Lewis and J. M. Haviland-Jones (Eds.) *Handbook of Emotions*, 2nd Ed. New York: Guilford Press, 253–264.

Kagan, D. (1995). *On the Origins of War*. New York: Doubleday.

Kagan, J. (1984). *The Nature of the Child*. New York: Basic Books.

Kaplan, L. (1986). *Adolescence: The Farewell to Childhood*. Northvale, NJ: Jason Aronson.

Katan, A. (1961). Some Thoughts about the Role of Verbalization in Early Childhood. *Psychoanalytic Study of the Child*, Vol. 16, 184–188.

Kazdin, A. (2000). *Psychotherapy for Children and Adolescents: Directions for Research and Practice*. NY: Oxford University Press.

Kazdin, A. (2005). *Parent Management Training*. NY: Oxford University Press.

Keenan, K. (2000). Emotion Dysregulation as a Risk Factor for Child Psychopthology. *Clinical Psychology: Science and Practice*, Vol. 7, No. 4, 418–434.

Keller, H. (1984). *Geraldine's Blanket*. New York: Greenwillow Books.

Kendall, P. C. (2006). Guiding Theory for Therapy with Children and Adolescents. In P. C. Kendall (Ed.) *Child and Adolescent Therapy*, 3rd Ed. New York: Guilford Press, 3–30.

Kendall, P. and Suveg, C. (2006). Treating Anxiety Disorders in Youth. In P. C. Kendall (Ed.) *Child and Adolescent Therapy*, 3rd Ed. New York: Guilford Press, 243–294.

Kendall, P. C., Aschenbrand, S. G., and Hudson, J. L. (2003). Child-Focused Treatment of Anxiety. In E. A. Kazdin and J. R. Weisz (Eds.) *Evidence-Based Psychotherapies for Children and Adolescents*. New York: Guilford Press, 81–100.

Kernberg, P. (1983). Borderline Conditions: Childhood and Adolescent Aspects. In K. Robson (Ed.) *The Borderline Child: Approaches to Etiology, Diagnosis, and Treatment*. New York: McGraw-Hill, 101–120.

Kindlon, D. and Thompson, M. (1999). *Raising Cain: Protecting the Emotional Life of Boys*. New York: Ballantine Books.

King, R. A. (1993). Cookies for the Emperor: The Multiple Functions of Play in the Analysis of an Early Adolescent Boy. In A. Solnit, D. Cohen, and P. Neubauer (Eds.) *The Many Meanings of Play: A Psychoanalytic Perspective*. New Haven, CT: Yale University Press, 135–155.

Kobak, R., Cassidy, J., Lyons-Ruth, K., and Ziv, Y. (2006). Attachment, Stress, and Psychopathology: A Developmental Pathways Model. In D. Cicchetti and D. Cohen (Eds.) *Developmental Psychopathology*, 2nd Ed. Hoboken, NJ: John Wiley and Sons, 333–369.

Kochanska, G. (2002). Committed Compliance, Moral Self, and Internalization: A Mediational Model. *Developmental Psychology*, Vol. 38, No. 3, 339–351.

Kohn, A. (1993). *Punished by Rewards: The Trouble with Gold Stars, Incentive Plans, A's and Other Bribes*. New York: Houghton Mifflin.

Kohut, H. (1959). Introspection, Empathy, and Psychoanalysis: An Examination of the Relationship between Mode of Observation and Theory. *Journal of the American Psychoanalytic Association*, Vol. 7, 459–483.

Kohut, H. (1966). Forms and Transformation of Narcissism. In P. Ornstein (Ed.) *The Search for the Self: Selected Writings of Heinz Kohut: 1950–1978*. Madison, CT: International Universities Press, 1978, 427–460. (Originally published in *Journal of the American Psychoanalytic Association*, Vol. 14, 243–272.)

Kohut, H. (1971). *The Analysis of the Self.* New York: International Universities Press.

Kohut, H. (1972). Thoughts on Narcissism and Narcissistic Rage. *Psychoanalytic Study of the Child,* Vol. 27, 360–400.

Kohut, H. (1977). *The Restoration of the Self.* New York: International Universities Press.

Kohut, H. (1982). Introspection, Empathy, and the Semi-circle of Mental Health. *International Journal of Psychoanalysis,* Vol. 63, 395–407.

Koren-Karie, N., Oppenheim, D., and Goldsmith, D. F. (2007). Keeping the Inner World of the Child in Mind: Using the Insightfulness Assessment with Mothers in a Therapeutic Preschool. In D. Oppenheim and D. F. Goldsmith (Eds.) *Attachment Theory in Clinical Work with Children.* New York: Guilford Press, 31–57.

Kovacs, M., Sherrill, J., George, C. J., Pollock, M., Tumuluru, R. V., and Ho, V. (2006). Contextual Emotion-Regulation Therapy for Childhood Depression: Description and Pilot Testing of a New Intervention. *Journal of the American Academy of Child and Adolescent Psychiatry,* Vol. 45, No. 8, 892–903.

Kramer, P. (2005). *Against Depression.* New York: Viking Press.

Krugman, P. (2008). Poverty Is Poison. *New York Times,* February 18, 2008.

Krystal, H. (1976). Affect Tolerance. *Annual of Psychoanalysis,* Vol. 3, 179–219.

Lazarus, A. A. and Fay, A. (1982). Resistance or Rationalization? A Cognitive-Behavioral Perspective. In P. L. Wachtel (Ed.) *Resistance: Psychodynamic and Behavioral Approaches.* New York: Plenum Press, 115–132.

Leahy, R. L. (2001). *Overcoming Resistance in Cognitive Therapy.* New York: Guilford Press.

Lear, J. (1992). Paper presented at Annual Retreat, Westchester Center for the Study of Psychoanalysis and Psychotherapy, Harriman, NY, March 1992.

Lemerise, E. A. and Dodge, K. A. (2000). The Development of Anger and Hostile Interactions. In M. Lewis and J. M. Haviland-Jones (Eds.) *Handbook of Emotions,* 2nd Ed. New York: Guilford Press, 594–606.

Levenson, R. W. (1994). Human Emotions: A Functionalist View. In P. Ekman and R. J. Davidson (Eds.) *The Nature of Emotion: Fundamental Questions.* New York: Oxford University Press, 123–126.

Levine, M. (1987). *Developmental Variation and Learning Disorders.* Cambridge, MA: Educators.

Levine, M. (2003). *The Myth of Laziness.* New York: Simon & Shuster.

LeVine, R. A. (1974). Parental Goals: A Cross-Cultural View. *Teacher's College Record,* Vol. 76, 226–239.

Lewis, H. B. (1971). *Shame and Guilt in Neurosis.* New York: International Universities Press.

Lewis, H. B. (1989). Some Thoughts on the Moral Emotions of Shame and Guilt. In L. Cirillo, B. Kaplan, and S. Werner (Eds.) *Emotions in Ideal Human Development.* Hillsdale, NJ: Lawrence Erlbaum Associates, 35–51.

Lewis, M. (2003). The Role of the Self in Shame. *Social Research,* Vol. 70, No. 4, *1181–1204.*

Lewis, M. D. and Douglas, L. (1998). A Dynamic Systems Approach to Cognition-Emotion Interactions in Development. In M. F. Mascolo and S. Griffin (Eds.) *What Develops in Emotional Development?* New York: Plenum Press, 159–188.

Li, H. C. W., Lopez, V., and Lee, L. I. (2007). Effects of Preoperative Therapeutic Play on Outcomes of School-Age Children Undergoing Day Surgery. *Research in Nursing and Health,* Vol. 30, No. 3, 320–332.

Lochman, J. E., Powell, N. R., Whidby, J. M., and Fitzgerald, D. P. (2006). Aggressive Children: Cognitive-Behavioral Assessment and Treatment. In P. C. Kendall (Ed.) *Child and Adolescent Therapy*, 3rd Ed. New York: Guilford Press, 33–81.

Lovinger, S. L. (1998). *Child Psychotherapy: From Initial Contact to Termination.* Northvale, NJ: Jason Aronson.

Maccoby, E. E. (2007). Historical Overview of Socialization Theory and Research. In J. E. Grusec and P. D. Hastings (Eds.) *Handbook of Socialization: Theory and Research.* New York: Guilford Press.

Maier, S. and Watkins, L. (1998). Cytokines for Psychologists: Implications of Bidirectional Immune-to-Brain Communication for Understanding Behavior, Mood, and Cognition. *Psychological Review*, Vol. 105, No. 1, 83–107.

Malatesta-Magai, C. (1991). Emotional Socialization: Its Role in Personality and Developmental Psychopathology. In D. Cicchetti and S. Toth (Eds.) *Internalizing and Externalizing Expressions of Dysfunction: Rochester Symposium on Developmental Psychopathology*, Vol. 2. Hillsdale, NJ: Lawrence Erlbaum Associates, 203–224.

March, J. S., Leonard, H. L., and Swedo, S. (1995). Obsessive-Compulsive Disorder. In J. S. March (Ed.) *Anxiety Disorders in Children and Adolescents.* New York: Guilford Press, 251–275.

Marston, S. (1990). *The Magic of Encouragement: Nurturing Your Child's Self-Esteem.* New York: William Morrow.

Mathelin, C. (1999). *Lacanian Psychotherapy with Children: The Broken Piano.* New York: Other Press.

Matzinger, P. (2003). The Danger Model: A Renewed Sense of Self. *Science*, Vol. 296, 301–308.

Mayer, J. D. and Salovey, P. (1997). What Is Emotional Intelligence? In P. Salovey and D. J. Sluyter (Eds.) *Emotional Development and Emotional Intelligence: Educational Implications.* New York: Basic Books, 3–31.

Meeks, J. (1970). Children Who Cheat at Games. *Journal of the Academy of Child Psychiatry*, Vol. 9: 157–170.

Menaker, T. (2001). *Evocation.* Paper presented at Annual Retreat, Westchester Center for the Study of Psychoanalysis and Psychotherapy, Harriman, NY, March 2001.

Miller, J.D. III (1996). *Using Self Psychology in Child Psychotherapy.* Northvale, NJ: Jason Aronson.

Miller, M. (1987). *My Grandmother's Cookie Jar.* Los Angeles, CA: Price, Stern, Sloan.

Miller, P. and Sperry, L. L. (1987). The Socialization of Anger and Aggression. *Merrill-Palmer Quarterly*, Vol. 33, No. 1, 1–31.

Mitchell, S. (1988). *Relational Concepts in Psychoanalysis.* Cambridge, MA: Harvard University Press.

Moustakis, C. (1997). *Relationship Play Therapy.* Northvale, NJ: Jason Aronson.

Mueller, C. M. and Dweck, C. S. (1998). Intelligence Praise Can Undermine Motivation and Performance. *Journal of Personality and Social Psychology*, Vol. 75, *33–52.*

Nelson, W. M., Finch, A. J., and Ghee, A. C. (2006). Anger Management with Children and Adolescents: Cognitive-Behavioral Therapy. In P. C. Kendall (Ed.) *Child and Adolescent Therapy*, 3rd Ed. New York: Guilford Press, 114–165.

Nichols, M. P. (2004). *Stop Arguing with Your Kids.* New York: Guilford Press.

Novick, K. and Novick, J. (1987). The Essence of Masochism. *Psychoanalytic Study of the Child*, Vol. 42, 353–384.

Nussbaum, M. (2001). *Upheavals of Thought: The Intelligence of Emotions*. New York: Cambridge University Press.

Ogilvie, D.M. (1987). The Undesired Self: A Neglected Variable in Personality Research. *Journal of Personality and Social Psychology,* Vol. 52, No. 2, 379–385.

Ohman, A. (2000). Fear and Anxiety: Evolutionary, Cognitive, and Clinical Perspectives. In M. Lewis and J. M. Haviland-Jones (Eds.) *Handbook of Emotions,* 2nd Ed. New York: Guilford Press, 573–593.

Oppenheim, D. and Goldsmith, D. F. (2007). *Attachment Theory in Clinical Work with Children*. New York: Guilford Press.

Oram, K. (2005). Boredom: Unprocessed Pain in the Treatment of a Narcissistic Boy and His Family. *Journal of Infant, Child, and Adolescent Psychotherapy*, Vol. 4, 233–243.

Ornstein, A. (1976). Making Contact with the Inner World of the Child: Toward a Theory of Psychoanalytic Psychotherapy with Children. *Comprehensive Psychiatry*, Vol. 17, No. 1, 3–36.

Osofsky, J. (1995). Applied Psychoanalysis: Research with Infants and Adolescents at High Risk Informs Psychoanalysis. In T. Shapiro and R. Emde (Eds.) *Research in Psychoanalysis: Process, Development, and Outcome.* Madison, CT: International Universities Press, 193–207.

Panksepp, J. (1998). *Affective Neuroscience*. Oxford: Oxford University Press.

Panksepp, J. (2001). The Long-Term Psychobiological Consequences of Infant Emotions: Prescriptions for the Twenty-first Century. *Infant Mental Health Journal*, Vol. 22, Nos. 1–2, 132–173.

Panksepp, J. (2007). *The Role of Play and Laughter in the Maturation of Pro-social Brains.* Paper presented at International Association of Neuro-psychoanalysis, New York, March 2007.

Panksepp, J. and Burgdorf, J. (2003). "Laughing" Rats and the Evolutionary Antecedents of Human Joy? *Physiology and Behavior*, Vol. 79, 533–547.

Parens, H. (1987). *Aggression in Our Children*. Northvale, NJ: Jason Aronson.

Parpal, M. and Maccoby, E. E. (1985). Maternal Responsiveness and Subsequent Child Compliance. *Child Development,* Vol. 56, 1326–1334.

Patterson, G. (1982). *Coercive Family Processes*. Eugene, OR: Castalia.

Phelan, T. W. (1995). *1-2-3 Magic: Effective Discipline for Children 2–12, 2nd Ed.* Glen Ellyn, IL: Child Management.

Pine, F. (1979). On the Expansion of the Affect Array. *Bulletin of the Meninger Clinic*, Vol. 43, No. 1, 79–95.

Pine, F. (1985). *Developmental Theory and Clinical Process*. New Haven, CT: Yale University Press.

Pollack, W. (1998). *Real Boys: Rescuing Our Sons from the Myths of Manhood*. New York: Henry Holt.

Powell, E. A. (1990). *Thomas Cole*. New York: Harry N. Abrams.

Rabian, B. and Bottjer, S. J. (2008). Sleep Problems. In A. Eisen (Ed.) *Treating Childhood Behavioral and Emotional Problems: A Step-by-Step, Evidence-Based Approach*. New York: Guilford Press, 365–410.

Reed, M. B. and Aspinwall, L. G. (1998). Self-Affirmation Reduces Biased Processing of Health-Risk Information. *Motivation and Emotion,* Vol. 22, No. 2, 99–132.

Reiss, S., Silverman, W., and Weems, C. (2001). Anxiety Sensitivity. In M. W. Vasey and M. R. Dadds (Eds.), *The Developmental Psychopathology of Anxiety*. New York: Oxford University Press, 92–111.

Reivich, K., Gillham, J. E., Chaplin, T. M., and Seligman, M. E. P. (2006). From Helplessness to Optimism. In R. Brooks and S. Goldstein (Eds.) *Handbook of Resilience in Children.* New York: Springer, 223–237.

Rizzolatti, G. and Arbib, M. A. (1998). Language within Our Grasp. *Trends Neuroscience,* Vol. 21, 188–194.

Russell, B. (1930). *The Conquest of Happiness.* London: Routledge Classics.

Saarni, C. (1997). Emotional Competence and Self-Regulation in Childhood. In P. Salovey and D. J. Sluyter (Eds.) *Emotional Development and Emotional Intelligence: Educational Implications.* New York: Basic Books, 35–66.

Sacks, O. (1973). *Awakenings.* New York: Random House.

Salovey, P. and Mayer, J. D. (1990). Emotional Intelligence. *Imagination, Cognition, and Personality,* Vol. 9, 185–211.

Sander, L. (2002). Thinking Differently: Principles of Process in Living Systems and the Specificity of Being Known. *Psychoanalytic Dialogues,* Vol. 12, No. 1, 11–43.

Sandler, J. and Sandler, A. M. (1998). *Internal Objects Revisited.* Madison, CT: International Universities Press.

Sapolsky, R. (1996). *Why Stress Is Bad for Your Brain.* Science, Vol. 273, 749–750.

Schafer, R. (1999). *My Search for the Heart of Psychoanalysis.* Paper presented at the Annual conference of the Westchester Center for the Study of Psychoanalysis and Psychotherapy, Tarrytown, NY, March 1999.

Scheff, T. J. (1998). Shame in the Labeling of Mental Illness. In P. Gilbert and B. Andrews (Eds.) *Shame: Interpersonal Behavior, Psychopathology, and Culture.* New York: Oxford University Press, 191–205.

Schore, A. N. (1994*). Affect Regulation and the Origin of the Self.* Hillsdale, NJ: Lawrence Erlbaum Associates.

Schore, A. N. (1998). Early Shame Experiences and Infant Brain Development. In P. Gilbert and B. Andrews (Eds.) *Shame: Interpersonal Behavior, Psychopathology, and Culture.* New York: Oxford University Press, 57–77.

Schwartz, J. (1996). *Brain Lock: Free Yourself from Obsessive-Compulsive Behavior.* New York: Regan Books.

Seligman, M. (1995). *The Optimistic Child.* Boston, MA: Houghton Mifflin.

Shapiro, T. (1983). The Unconscious Still Occupies Us. *Psychoanalytic Study of the Child,* Vol. 38, 547–568.

Shapiro, T. and Esman, A, (1985). Psychotherapy with Children and Adolescents: Still Relevant in the 1980s? *Psychiatric Clinics of North America,* Vol. 8, No. 4, 909–921.

Siegel, D. and Hartzell, M. (2003). *Parenting from the Inside Out.* New York: Penguin Putnam.

Silvia, P. J. (2005). What is Interesting? Exploring the Appraisal Structure of Interest. *Emotion,* Vol. 5, No. 1, 89–102.

Singer, D. G. (1993). *Playing for Their Lives: Helping Troubled Children through Play Therapy.* New York: Free Press.

Singer, D. G. and Singer, J. L. (2005). *Imagination and Play in the Electronic Age.* Cambridge, MA: Harvard University Press.

Slade, A. (1994). Making Meaning and Making Believe: Their Role in the Clinical Process. In A. Slade and D. P. Wolf (Eds.) *Children at Play.* New York: Oxford University Press, 87–110.

Slade, A. (1999). Representation, Symbolization, and Affect Regulation in the Concomitant Treatment of a Mother and Child: Attachment Theory and Child Psychotherapy. *Psychoanalytic Inquiry,* Vol. 19, 797–830.

Slade, A. (2002). Moments of Regulation and the Development of Self-Narratives. *Journal of Infant, Child, and Adolescent Psychotherapy*, Vol. 2, No. 4, 1–10.

Slade, A. (2006). Reflective Parenting Programs: Theory and Development. *Psychoanalytic Inquiry*, Vol. 4 September/October, 2006, 640–657.

Smith, H. (2003). Conceptions of Conflict in Psychoanalytic Theory and Practice. *Psychoanalytic Quarterly*, Vol. LXXII, No. 1, 49–96.

Sorce, J. and Emde, R. (1981). Mother's Presence Is Not Enough: The Effect of Emotional Availability on Infant Exploration. *Developmental Psychology*, Vol. 17, 737–745.

Spiegel, S. (1996). *An Interpersonal Approach to Child and Adolescent Psychotherapy.* Northvale, NJ: Jason Aronson.

Spillius, E. B. (1997). Varieties of Envious Experience. In R. Schafer (Ed.) *The Contemporary Kleinians of London.* Madison, CT: International Universities Press, 143–171.

Sroufe, L. A., Carlson, E. A., Levy, A. K., and Egeland, B. (1999). Implications of Attachment Theory for Developmental Psychopathology. *Development and Psychopathology*, Vol. 11, 1–13.

Sroufe, L. A., Egeland, B., Carlson, E. A., and Collins, W. A. (2005). *The Development of the Person.* New York: Guilford Press.

Stark, K. D., Hargrave, J., Hersh, B., Greenberg, M., Herren, J., and Fisher, M. (2008). Treatment of Childhood Depression: The Action Treatment Program. In J. R. Z. Abela and B. L. Hankin (Eds.) *Handbook of Depression in Children and Adolescents.* New York: Guilford Press.

Stern, D. (1985). *The Interpersonal World of the Infant.* New York: Basic Books.

Stipek, D. (1995). The Development of Pride and Shame in Toddlers. In J. P. Tangney and K. W. Fischer (Eds.) *Self-Conscious Emotions: The Psychology of Shame, Guilt, Embarrassment, and Pride.* New York: Guilford Press, 237–252.

Sugarman, A. (1994). Toward Helping Child Analysands Observe Mental Functioning. *Psychoanalytic Psychology*, Vol. 2, No. 3, 329–341.

Sugarman, A. (2003). A New Model for Conceptualizing Insightfulness in the Psychoanalysis of Young Children. *Psychoanalytic Quarterly*, Vol. LXXII, No. 2, 325–355.

Sullivan, H. S. (1953). *The Interpersonal Theory of Psychiatry.* New York: W. W. Norton.

Suth, R. B. (1996). A Self-Psychological Approach to Child Therapy: A Case Study. In A. Goldberg (Ed.) *Basic Ideas Reconsidered: Progress in Self Psychology*, Vol. 12. Hillsdale, NJ: Analytic Press.

Swedo, S. E., Leonard, H. L., Garvey, M., Mittleman, B., Allen, A.J., Perlmutter, S., Lougee, L., Dow, S., Zamkoff, J., and Dubbert, B. K. (1998). Pediatric Autoimmune Neuropsychiatric Disorders Associated with Streptococcal Infections: Clinical Description of the First 50 Cases. *American Journal of Psychiatry*, Vol. 155, 2, 265–271.

Taffel, R. (2001). *Getting Through to Difficult Kids and Parents.* New York: Guilford Press.

Thompson, R. A., Laible, D. J., and Ontai, L. L. (2003). Early Understandings of Emotion, Morality, and Self: Developing a Working Model. *Advances in Child Development and Behavior*, Vol. 31, 137–171.

Toth, S. and Cicchetti, D. (1999). Developmental Psychopathology and Child Psychotherapy. In S. W. Russ and T. H. Ollendick (Eds.) *Handbook of Psychotherapies with Children and Families.* New York: Plenum Publishers, 15–44.

Tronick, E. Z. (1989). Emotions and Emotional Communication in Infants. *American Psychologist*, Vol. 44, 112–119.

Tronick, E. Z. (2006). The Inherent Stress of Normal Daily Life and Social Interaction Leads to the Development of Coping and Resilience, and Variation in Resilience in Infants and Young Children: Comments on the Papers of Suomi and Klebanov & Brooks-Gunn. In M. Lester, A. Masten, and B. McEwan (Eds.) *Resilience in Children. Annals of the New York Academy of Sciences,* Vol. 1094, 83–104.

Tyson, P. (1998). Developmental Roots of Adolescent Disturbance. In A. Esman (Ed.) *Adolescent Psychiatry,* Vol. 23, 21–39.

Tyson, P. and Tyson, R. L. (1990). *Psychoanalytic Theories of Development.* New Haven, CT: Yale University Press.

Volkan, V. D. (1988). *The Need to Have Enemies and Allies: From Clinical Practice to International Relationships.* Northvale, NJ: Jason Aronson.

Wachs, T. D. (2006). Contributions of Temperament to Buffering and Sensitization Processes in Children's Development. In M. Lester, A. Masten, and B. McEwan (Eds.) *Resilience in Children. Annals of the New York Academy of Sciences,* Vol. 1094, 28–39.

Wachtel, E. (2001). The Language of Becoming: Helping Children Change How They Think about Themselves. *Family Process,* Vol. 40, No. 4, 369–383.

Watson, J. B. (1928). *Psychological Care of Infant and Child.* New York: W. W. Norton.

Webster-Stratton, C. and Reid. M. J. (2003). The Incredible Years Parents, Teachers, and Children Training Series: A Multifaceted Treatment Approach for Young Children with Conduct Problems. In E. A. Kazdin and J. R. Weisz (Eds.) *Evidence-Based Psychotherapies for Children and Adolescents.* New York: Guilford Press, 224–240.

Weisfeld, G. E. (1997). Discrete Emotions Theory with Specific Reference to Pride and Shame. In N. L. Segal, G. Weisfeld, and C. C. Weisfeld (Eds.) *Uniting Psychology and Biology: Integrative Perspectives in Human Development.* Washington, DC: American Psychological Association.

Werner, E. (1995). Resilience in Development. *Current Directions in Psychological Science,* Vol. 4, No. 3, 81–85.

Winnicott, D. W. (1956/1975). The Antisocial Tendency. In D. W. Winnicott, *Through Paediatrics to Psycho-analysis.* New York: Basic Books.

Winnicott, D. W. (1960/1965). Ego Distortion in Terms of True and False Self. In *The Maturational Processes and the Facilitating Environment.* New York: International Universities Press, 140–152.

Winnicott, D. W. (1963/1965). The Development of the Capacity for Concern. In *The Maturational Processes and the Facilitating Environment.* New York: International Universities Press, 73–82.

Wright, L., Everett, F., and Roisman, L. (1986). *Experiential Psychotherapy with Children.* Baltimore, MD: Johns Hopkins University Press.

Wyman, P. A., Cowen, E. L., Work, W. C., and Kerley, J. H. (1993). The Role of Children's Future Expectations in Self-System Functioning and Adjustment to Life Stress: A Prospective Study of Urban At-Risk Children. *Development and Psychopathology,* 5: 649–661.

Yankelovich, D. (1999). *The Magic of Dialogue: Transforming Conflict into Cooperation.* New York: Simon & Shuster.

Yanof, J.A. (1996). Language, Communication and Transference in Child Analysis. *Journal of the American Psychoanalytic Association,* Vol. 44, No.1, 79–116.

Zetzel, E. (1965). *The Capacity for Emotional Growth.* New York: International Universities Press.

Index

CPSIA information can be obtained
at www.ICGtesting.com
Printed in the USA
LVOW12*0724150817
545076LV00006B/21/P

9 780195 366860